D1477967

AIRWISE

By the same author
The Curse of Icarus
Why Flying Endangers Your Health

Farrol S. Kahn

AIRWISE

The Essential Guide for Frequent Flyers

Index compiled by
Lyn Greenwood

SAFFRON WALDEN
THE C.W. DANIEL COMPANY LIMITED

First published in Great Britain in 1993
by The C.W. Daniel Company Limited
1 Church Path, Saffron Walden
Essex, CB10 1JP, England

ISBN 0 85207 264 3

This book is printed on
part-recycled paper

Disclaimer
Every effort has been made to ensure that the
information presented in this book is accurate.
Advice from a book has its limitations however,
and cannot always take into account the specific
circumstances of each individual passenger.
Any advice offered here is not intended to
replace counsel given by competent medical
personnel. If you have a problem consult your
physician or GP.

Designed and Produced by
Book Production Consultants plc, Cambridge
Typeset in Melior by
Rowland Phototypesetting Limited,
Bury St Edmunds, Suffolk
and printed and bound in the UK by
J. E. C. Potter & Son Limited, Stamford, Lincs.

Dedication

To my dear wife from 'across the line' and my daughters, Tasha and Pippa.

Acknowledgements
I wish to thank two precursors of my book. The first is Professor John Bell of the University of Oxford, who provided me with the concept for my jetlag experiment. The second is Ian Miller whose enthusiasm was opportune at the embryonic state.

I am also indebted to Dr F. John Mills, Vice-President of Besselaar Associates and Professor D.A. Warrell, University of Oxford for the useful suggestions about the manuscript.

Others who have been most helpful include Maggie E. Anderson, Angela Baker, Captain Harry Bucknall, Archie Clowes, Chris Farley, Ann Dickson-Brown, Michael Edwards, Pat Evans, David Flanagan, Ken Fletcher, R. Gelder, John Hewitt, Dr Mike Hobbs, Chris Maclaren, John Muirhead, Carol Moss, Kathy O'Brien, David O'Neill, Alison Plummer, Arlette M. Robertson, Dr David R. Shlim, Lindsay Sandison, Tim Ward and Udo Wolf.

CONTENTS

	Introduction	1
CHAPTER ONE	Physiological Stressors of Flying	3
CHAPTER TWO	The Flight Environment	13
CHAPTER THREE	The Fearful Flyer	24
CHAPTER FOUR	How to Overcome Jetlag	34
CHAPTER FIVE	Immunization of Travellers	45
CHAPTER SIX	Airport Environment	49
CHAPTER SEVEN	Food, Drink and Advice	52
CHAPTER EIGHT	High Risk Conditions	57
CHAPTER NINE	The Armchair Aviator	68
	Destinations of High Altitude	74
	List of Approved Dosimetry Services	76
	Checklist of Vaccinations and Health Precautions	79
	Bibliography	82
	Index	84

INTRODUCTION

Airwise, the term and the title of the book both require a definition.

The term is easy to explain for it derives from the same notion as the word, streetwise. To be familiar with the ways of modern urban life, you need to know essential facts and use them to your benefit.

For example, if you want to be safe in New York (as in any other big city in the U.S. for that matter), do the following: Always walk fast, never make eye contact with strangers, give the impression at all times that you know where you are going (even if you do not), and above all, avoid dangerous neighbourhoods.

Airwise, in a similar manner, is to be familiar with the flight environment, on the ground and in the air, to your own advantage. If you want to be healthy and you fly a lot, there is a simple course of action to take: Be frugal with your intake of food and alcohol, excessive in the amount of water you drink, and on longhaul flights your behaviour should be contradictory. In the air, you should go into a state of semi-hibernation and on the ground in transit, exercise well.

As a title, *Airwise* ranges wide. It shows you why alcohol is more potent in the air than on the ground, and how you need never suffer from jetlag again if you have a basic understanding of cabin pressurization and air-conditioning. It provides you with an instant knowledge on how to survive a crash, how to take the fear out of flying and what to do in a decompression – when the cabin pressure fails.

At the heart of the book though is health. Did you know that there are high risk conditions which prevent you from flying? These vary from asthma, bronchitis, stomach ulcers to angina, high blood pressure and recent surgery – you should wait at least 10 days even after the removal of your tonsils before you fly. To know whether you are on a high risk list or not, your G.P. or Physician should complete a medical information form for the airlines.

Also, it is essential for frequent flyers to have a medical examination once a year with an aviation specialist. This is due to the fact that a passenger's body is subject to five physiological stressors every flight.

Issues too are raised in the book. Of these, radiation is one of the most significant. Although aircrew are now classified by the National Radiological Protection Board as being a group exposed to higher levels than normal of radiation, frequent flyers are not. This is in spite of the fact that the latter do the same amount of, if not more, flying hours. As a result, these passengers exceed the maximum permissible dosage and are unprotected as a group. The other issue is smoking which should be banned on all flights because not only are the passengers exposed to carcinogens in tobacco smoke, but it also deprives them of oxygen in the cabin through the presence of carbon monoxide.

Exalted subjects too are included. Socrates's brief discourse on flying and poetry which lauds the miracle of flight.

In all, *Airwise* provides the reader with gobbets of air wisdom which are readily absorbed on board where attention spans are short. But this book is written mostly for those who like to have their cake and eat it. For them, New York is just across the street from London or Tokyo and they cross those streets many times in a week or month. They will fly anywhere for business, to play sport, to perform at concerts or negotiate political settlements. Like Henry Kissinger aka 'Super K' they will travel 24,230 miles on 41 flights in 34 days. However, now they can do it without having a bypass or angina.

CHAPTER ONE

PHYSIOLOGICAL STRESSORS OF FLYING

There are five physiological stressors of flying:
1. Less air to breathe including oxygen;
2. Air expands in cavities or semi-cavities of the body;
3. Extreme dry air causes rapid moisture loss;
4. Air is polluted through smoking, inadequate ventilation and recycling systems.
5. Doses of radiation.

The human factor has always taken a back seat in aviation. It is understandable because when heavier-than-air flying machines were first developed, the biggest problem was to keep them up long enough safely. Therefore, engineering has been preoccupied with the aircraft at the expense of the passengers who fly in it.

This does not mean that the health and fitness of the pilot (the airline or military) is neglected. On the contrary, they are well cared for by aviation specialists who play a supporting role in aviation. This is essential because the modern aircraft is a compromise between the ideal atmosphere on the ground and the hostile atmosphere at high altitude. In a nutshell, the cabin environment is artificial and is designated as our life support system. As a result, there are risks to our bodies whether we are fit or not.

To gain insight into what we are up against, I have to introduce the 'Father of Aviation Medicine', Paul Bert (1833–1866). He was a French doctor and physiologist who did experiments to determine what happens to the body at high altitudes.

What Bert did was unique. He built the world's first pressure chamber and was able to simulate conditions at various altitudes. Essentially, the chamber consisted of two boilers, 6½ feet high and 3¼ feet in diameter, connected by a door and with portholes, through which he could view subjects in the vacuum created by a steam-driven pump. There were two barometers – a large one outside the boilers and one inside, which enabled him to determine the pressure in the chamber. By withdrawing the air, he could achieve the maximum equivalent of up to 36,000 ft or 3 psi (pounds per square inch).

He could therefore demonstrate the effects of a decrease in pressure (or a deficiency of air) and an increase in the volume of air on the body. For that is what occurs when you ascend. The converse is the true when you descend. It is known as Boyle's Law, and was discovered by Robert Boyle (1627–1691).

In experiments with large dogs, who were taken 'up' to 28,000 ft, Bert noticed that with decreased pressure, the heart and respiration rate increased. The digestion slowed down and intestinal gases expanded. Body temperature dropped and the dogs became dull and listless. If they were taken 'up' too fast, there was paralysis of the hind quarters and the subjects died.

As an intrepid physiologist, Bert experimented on himself too. He was of average height, 5 ft 7 in, weight, 140 lbs, and aged about 40, when he carried them out. On one occasion, he was at 8,000 feet and on another, reached 16,000 feet. He noticed an increase in his pulse from 58 at sea level to 63 at 8,000 feet and between 76–80 at 16,000 feet, which is where he began to inhale oxygen. On the way 'up' he experienced nausea, he had trouble with his vision, his stomach became distended and gas escaped from his mouth and anus. Other symptoms he noticed were dizziness, headache, uncontrollable trembling in his legs and congestion in his head.

Here then are two physiological stressors of flying.

1. Hypoxia or oxygen lack

Whenever we travel on an aircraft, we all suffer from a condition known as mild hypoxia. This is defined as a decrease below normal levels of oxygen in the air, blood or tissues. The reason is quite simple. The cabin altitude controller is set at between 6,000–8,000 feet and as a result, there is 20–26% less oxygen (partial pressure) to breathe.

An analogous condition that most people, particularly skiers and climbers, will be more familiar with is mountain sickness. The central feature is hypoxia, with cold and exercise as contributory factors. However, it can be prevented if sufficient time is taken to acclimatise to the altitude or if the sufferer at the onset simply descends. The same is true of mild hypoxia for when we leave the aircraft the condition disappears. The symptoms of acute hypoxia were described by the well-known physiologist, Joseph Barcroft, in 1920, as similar to alcoholic intoxication – headache, mental confusion, drowsiness, muscular weakness and lack of coordination. These may be accompanied by singing or shouting, a feeling of satisfaction and a sense of power.

In the case of mild hypoxia, there is a small increase in the heart and breathing rate and a slight interference in the brain's functions. As a result, the symptoms include headaches, mental blocks, dizzy spells, fatigue, a sensation of looking without seeing and mental and physical impairments. These effects are partly a consequence of the body juggling with lesser amounts of oxygen and deciding which part gets what proportion. Under normal circumstances, the heart consumes 11% of the oxygen intake, the brain 18%, the kidney 7%, the intestines 25%, the skeletal muscle 30%, the skin 2% and the other organs 7%.

What may surprise people is that some of the symptoms usually attributed to jetlag are in fact the result of hypoxia. In experiments carried out by the R.A.F. Institute of Aviation Medicine, it was found that a mild degree of oxygen lack causes people to tire more easily and to learn or do new tasks less quickly. The drinking of alcohol, smoking or inhaling tobacco smoke or over-breathing tend to increase your hypoxia. If you do not feel well on board, you can always ask for supplemental oxygen as all airlines carry portable canisters of the gas.

2. The balloon body

Passengers swell during the flight. The expansion of gas inflates the cavities such as the alimentary canal, ears and sinuses. If you have a small amount of air in your stomach – say 100 ml, according to Boyle's Law, it will increase by 25% at 6,000 ft cabin altitude and by 35% at 8,000 ft cabin pressure.

As a result, the abdomen will tend to press up against the diaphragm and in turn can cause it to press up against a fatty or slightly diseased heart. This occurs particularly when restrictive clothing of any kind is worn. The consequent discomfort will be often mistaken by the passenger or cabin staff for angina. (The pain is usually manifested over the breastbone.) By this time, the passenger is panicking and has started to hyperventilate, becoming short of breath. Soon the passenger becomes grey, sweaty and will probably faint.

Sometimes, he or she may become 'airsick' or vomit on descent or soon after landing. This may be caused by the 135 ml of gas which has shrunk rapidly to 100 ml, and the stomach walls follow the outline of the contents and keep on contracting – producing vomiting even after landing. The body is a balloon.

Other cases where trapped gas can cause problems in flight include:

a. Teeth
Changes in cabin pressure can cause toothache. It is advisable to see your dentist if you have any loose fillings or abscesses.

b. Ears and Sinuses

The middle ear is the air-filled space between the eardrum and the inner ear. The only access of air to the middle ear is through the eustachian tube that opens at the back of the throat, and in the case of the sinuses, there are tiny holes called ostia that vent into the back of the nose.

Under normal circumstances, the air can expand and contract without difficulty. However, during a head cold, for example, the lining of the eustachian tube and the nasal sinuses become swollen and inflamed. It is then painful to vent air. Aircrew are usually grounded temporarily if they have colds. The use of a decongestant spray is advisable if you fly. In some instances, the ear drum may be perforated and, if the descent or ascent is sudden, dizziness and disorientation, termed 'pressure vertigo' can occur. In other instances, passengers may suffer from temporary deafness or tinnitus – a ringing in the ears – for a week or fortnight later.

c. Surgery

Whenever the skin is cut, such as in an operation, or the interior wall of the uterus or cervix is scraped in a curettage, air is introduced into the wound. The air needs time to be reabsorbed – anything from a week to a month – depending on the type of surgery. Therefore, you should not fly before this period. Otherwise, the trapped air will expand and may cause a haemorrhage.

d. Plaster Casts

Consider splitting the cast before a flight, particularly if the skin underneath is still swollen. The trapped gas in the plaster may compress the limb. The combination of vascular compression and a degree of oxygen lack has been known to cause gangrene following longhaul flights.

After some 670 experiments with people and animals, Paul Bert concluded that all organisms on earth are acclimatized to air (oxygen) at sea level. Any increase or decrease may be harmful to them.

It is a short step from the pressure chamber to the pressurised cabin in which we usually fly. Instead of the air being withdrawn in the chamber, it is compressed to fill the cabin. The altitudes reached at cruise level in the aircraft vary from 5,000 to 8,000 feet.

It is one thing to simulate conditions of flying on the ground as Dr Bert did and another to conduct a study under real conditions in the air. Over the past 60 years, this has been carried out by flight surgeons, scientists and medical researchers mainly in the armed forces. As a result, numerous textbooks on aviation and later aerospace medicine have been written.

Of the other physiological stressors, two are derived from the imperfections of the aircraft's environmental control system, and the fifth is a high altitude health hazard.

3. Dry air or dehydration

The air that enters an aircraft at 35,000 ft plus is drier than any desert on earth. The water content falls from 10 g/kg at sea level to 0.15 g/kg of dry air at high altitude. In terms of relative humidity it is around 1% compared with 25% which is found in a centrally heated room. Both A.S.H.R.A.E. (Association of Heating, Refrigeration and Air-Conditioning Engineers) and N.I.O.S.H. (National Institute for Occupational Safety and Health) have indicated that the comfort zone should be between 30–65% relative humidity.

Water is an essential ingredient of our bodies and ranks second only to air as the most urgent of the body's needs. It accounts for 50–60% of the adult's weight and children have smaller reserves than adults. In the case of a minor deficiency through not drinking enough, the result is dry skin, pasty appearance and constipation. Dehydration can also exacerbate irritation from other pollutants in the lungs, nose and throat.

On board, it is insidious because you do not

8

sweat nor do you feel thirsty as you would in the heat on the ground. Nevertheless, any moisture is rapidly removed by evaporation as it is formed. If you want to prevent dry skin, it is more beneficial to use a gel or moisturiser rather than a spray. Most of the water content in the latter evaporates and little penetrates the skin.

To have a humidifier on an aircraft for passengers would be costly because of the weight penalty of the water. The only other way of boosting the relative humidity is to have a high load factor. The resultant moisture from passengers' breath and perspiration can increase the relative humidity from 1% to 10–20% or more.

4. The stale brewed air

For years flight attendants have protested over the quality of air found in the cabin environment. Their main concern has been tobacco smoke, a known carcinogen, and they have been partly successful as smoking bans have been instituted on some domestic and international flights. However, there is a good case for banning smoking altogether on board because it increases the effect of another physiological stressor, the lack of oxygen.

The carbon monoxide in environmental tobacco smoke forms carboxyhaemoglobin in the blood which prevents it from carrying oxygen to the tissues. The gas, which is a constituent of motor vehicle exhaust, is favoured by suicides who connect a hose to carry it into the vehicle and asphyxiate themselves. As a result, the oxygen deficiency of 20–26% experienced by the passenger is further increased by 5–10% through the presence of tobacco smoke.

Smokers and aircrew working in the smoking area of an aircraft with a cabin altitude of about 8,000 feet can have an effective oxygen saturation level as low as 83–85%. In hospitals patients with oxygen saturation levels below 85% are cause for concern. Yet this condition occurs in commercial aircraft among passengers and crew members.

9

Although most passengers will not be affected by these levels, those over 50 years of age, with limited cardiorespiratory capacity due to age, overweight or disease may experience symptoms of nausea, dizziness, shortness of breath or chest pains. Dizziness in fact is the most common medical problem on board major airlines. There is little doubt that smoking should be banned on all flights.

Other components of the brew include: ozone, a gas that is a strong oxidising agent similar to chlorine and is found at high altitude; an excess of carbon dioxide which is produced by human breathing and dry ice in the inflight galleys, and can affect some heart conditions; viruses, bacteria and fungi that spread contagious diseases and allergies; and aerosols from plastics used on board.

The problem of polluted air can be solved by not recirculating stale air and the use of filters to remove contaminants.

5. Cosmic radiation

Whenever you fly at high altitude, you are exposed to greater radiation doses than you would on the ground. Contrary to what some people believe, the airframes do not protect passengers from radiation. The dose depends on altitude and it varies from 100–200 times more. The Concorde, for example, which cruises at 60,000 ft, has a dose rate per hour of twice that of a subsonic like a Boeing 747. But then it flies twice as fast so the radiation exposures for both types of aircraft are about the same.

The National Radiological Protection Board (N.R.P.B.), an independent institution which advises the Government, recommends a maximum dosage of 15 millisieverts (mSv) per year for occupational exposures and 0.3 mSv per year for members of the public. Workers in the nuclear industry are classed as occupationally exposed individuals. The exposure levels vary from a total average of 4.5 mSv to 15 mSv. Their health therefore is closely monitored for non-fatal cancers, fatal cancers and hereditary effects of radiation, and includes the use of thermoluminescent personal dosemeters (T.L.D.), regular medicals and blood counts.

Aircrew too, according to the N.R.P.B. fit into the category of occupational radiation and are on a par with nuclear workers. Accordingly, their health is monitored by the Civil Aviation Authority. However, this is mainly based on the limited amount of hours that can be spent by the flight crew in the air. There is a maximum of 900 hours per year, but in practice it is nearer 600–700 hours. Of the 20,000 aircrew in the U.K., 19,900 receive 4.5 mSv and 100 between 5–15 mSv. The latter are pilots who fly Concorde or transpolar routes.

Frequent flyers can spend an average of between 5 and 15 hours or more in the air per week. Such radiation exposure, 3.23 mSv to 4.5 mSv, places them in the same category as workers in the medical, dental, veterinary, industrial radiography, mining (coal and non-coal) and nuclear industries. However, as they are not officially recognised as occupationally exposed individuals, they are exceeding the maximum permissible dosage for members of the public by up to 10–15 times. The dosage will vary in individuals as it will not only depend on the number of hours flown per annum but on whether flights were taken during periods of solar radiation or over transpolar routes.

Although the risk of inducing a fatal cancer over 10 years with a total dose of 50 mSv is low, of 100,000 frequent flyers, there is a probability that 200 will die of a fatal cancer. This should be compared to the natural risk of death from cancer which is around 1 in 4 or 25,000 out of 100,000.

Some people may consider it prudent to begin monitoring their doses immediately and before such action is recommended by the N.R.P.B. This can be done through an approved dosimetery laboratory which will provide a thermoluminescent dosemeter (T.L.D.) or a film badge (a list is supplied in the appendix). Alternatively,

11

you can monitor your own radiation doses with a direct reading personal dosemeter (costing about £250) which contains its own geiger counter and can be worn much like a fountain pen.

Of the organs or tissues most likely to be at risk are the reproductive organs, followed by red bone marrow, colon, lung and stomach. However, the greatest risk is to the foetus and once pregnancy is declared, particularly in the first three months, exposure to radiation should be restricted.

Several research projects have shown that all types of childhood cancer and leukemia are doubled by extremely small doses of radiation. Pregnant frequent flyers, couriers or flight attendants should reduce the amount of flying, avoid the polar routes and periods of intense solar activity, or stop flying during the trimester of their pregnancy.

For fit passengers, the five physiological stressors add to the strain on the body which in turn compensates for them. For the unfit passengers, it is another matter. They can be tipped over into the critical phase of their illness.

CHAPTER TWO

THE FLIGHT ENVIRONMENT

The Aircraft Cabin

The higher a plane flies, the faster it travels because the air is thinner at altitude and offers less resistance than the thicker air at sea level. For example, the pressure of air at sea level is 14 lb/square inch (760 mmHg), but at 40,000 ft it is 2.7 lb/square inch (141 mmHg) and is 1 lb/square inch (54 mmHg) at 60,000 ft. Concorde, which cruises at altitudes of 50,000–60,000 ft has a speed of over 2 Mach (1,320 mph). Other commercial aircraft travel at speeds of about 500 mph at an altitude of 30,000–40,000 ft. However, if passengers were exposed to such low pressure they would be unconscious within seconds and dead several minutes later from lack of oxygen.

Therefore, whenever aircraft operate at high altitude, the cabins have to be pressurised. At cruise level, those pressures can vary from 12.2–10.8 psi which is an equivalent altitude of 5,000–8,000 ft. The optimum cabin altitude is 8,000 ft and, if due to a malfunction, the altitude rises to 10,000 ft, a warning message flashes on and a siren sounds in the cockpit.

The air that is used to pressurise the cabin is bled from the jet engines where it is not only under great pressure but very hot. After being cooled in a heat exchanger, the bleed air is fed into the fuselage from the front to the rear where it is expelled through one-way valves. However, three-quarters of the bled air passes through the air conditioning system and as a result, bleed and conditioned air is mixed before being expelled at the rate of about every three minutes.

There are three air conditioning packs on a

13

Boeing 747 and the cabin air flows at the rate of 6,000 cubic feet a minute (C.F.M.). While the flight crew in the cockpit get as much as 60–150 C.F.M. of air per person, and the First Class passengers – between 30–50 C.F.M., the Economy Class passengers and flight attendants can get as little as 7–10 C.F.M. The flight crew also have the additional benefit of humidifiers so that they can perform their duties with minimum discomfort or fatigue.

Whenever air is bled from the engine, the thrust is reduced and the pilot uses more fuel to compensate for this loss. To save on fuel consumption, one air conditioning unit is usually shut down once proper pressure and temperature is reached. Another method of reducing fuel costs is to recirculate 50% of the air through the installation of recirculation fans (there are four on the 747-400) and to expel it once every 12 minutes.

Cabin pressure or altitude is controlled by regulating the discharge of the mixed air through outflow valves at the rear of the aircraft while the airframe has to be strong enough to withstand a pressurisation of some 9 pounds/square inch at cruising height.

Decompression

The problems of altitude, ie mainly the danger of hypoxia, become apparent when there is a failure of pressurization or, as it is known, a decompression.

What happens in a decompression? The same that occurs when a rubber balloon which is filled with air bursts or deflates if the neck is not held tightly. Air rushes out either rapidly or slowly.

Should the decompression be the result of a hole or crack in the aircraft, then the suction is so great that it can pull passengers out of their seatbelts. There was the case of a British Airways pilot who was sucked out of the cockpit when a window dropped from its frame. He was saved because members of the aircrew hung onto his legs until the aircraft had landed safely.

Two other signs of a decompression are a loud

bang that is followed by a noise of rushing icy, cold air and the misting of everything, and the appearance of oxygen masks from the ceiling. The other cause of decompression is the malfunction of the air conditioning system. This can happen, for example, when components have been affected by a build-up of nicotine tar. The tar has to be scraped out of the air ducts regularly.

It is essential to act quickly in a decompression as it is an emergency. Reach for a mask immediately, and breathe oxygen. If necessary, tug at the tubing to initiate the supply.

Also expect the aircraft to go into a dive as the pilot takes evasive action. This can complicate the handling of the oxygen mask as the steep angle of descent forces the passenger forward. Backward facing seats would prevent such movement.

Once you have secured your own supply, assist others like children with attaching their mask. After the event, make sure that you are examined by an aviation medical specialist. This is important as you may be affected for days or even weeks later.

Sick Aircraft Syndrome

The environmental control system (E.C.S.) found on an aircraft is not dissimilar to a heating, ventilating and air conditioning (H.V.A.C.) system found in modern sealed buildings, and is subject to similar contaminants and pollutants.

The term, a sick building, which is related to ventilation, air tightness and unhygienic water systems, can also be applied to an aircraft. For not only is there a trend towards recycling more stale air (up to 50% in new aircraft) but to contravene health regulations that apply to confined environments on the ground.

If there is inadequate ventilation and poor filtration, microbes causing allergic and infectious diseases are allowed to build up in stagnant air to unacceptable levels. In the case of carbon dioxide, the standards in buildings are 1,000 parts per million by volume (p.p.m.v.). However, it has been found to be as high as 5,000 p.p.m. on some U.S. airlines or 2,500 p.p.m.v. on a European airline which was operating air conditioning packs at 50% capacity. An excess of CO_2 can cause arrhythmias in passengers with heart conditions.

Although ozone (O_3) is not found on the ground, the Federal Aviation Administration established that the concentration level at altitudes of 32,000 ft should not exceed 0.25 p.p.m.v. During a period when these levels were monitored, 11% violated the limits. Ozone is a strong oxidising agent and is toxic to humans. Exposure to the gas can cause asthmatic symptoms and eye, nose and throat irritations, impair night vision and has a similar effect on chromosomes as x-rays. Ozone concentrations peak in the Northern Hemisphere during February to May.

The low levels of relative humidity, cosmic radiation and environmental tobacco smoke have already been dealt with in Chapter One. In the latter case, on some flights, tobacco smoke pours out of air ducts soon after take-off. Whether this demonstrates the ineffectiveness of the air conditioning equipment or the effectiveness of the recirculation fans is another matter.

The transmission rate of infectious or contagious diseases in the air, according to the U.S. Federal Center for Disease Control, may be as high as 72%. Influenza is a case in point. The density of passengers on board a tightly sealed aircraft combined with inadequate ventilation makes the flight environment ideal for the spread of fungi, viruses and bacteria.

When a plane was grounded in Alaska for three hours, without any fresh outside ventilation, there was an outbreak of influenza. A Canadian study demonstrated that microbes which had been released in the rear of an empty Boeing 707 contaminated 100% of the cabin. There have also been a couple of cases of atypical pneumonia which doctors believe have been caught on aircraft.

Aircraft ventilation rates in the Economy Class

are below the minimum standards of 20 cubic feet a minute (C.F.M.) recommended by the American Society of Heating and Refrigeration and Air Conditioning Engineers (A.S.H.R.A.E.) for indoor spaces on the ground. As was shown earlier, the rate of 7–10 C.F.M. is lower than that for First Class passengers and for the flight crew.

Is there an instant antidote for the Sick Aircraft Syndrome? Yes. Increase the ventilation rate. At a stroke we would reduce the levels of most of the pollutants. The disadvantages would be that the relative humidity would still be low and the concentration of ozone would be high. However, the latter can be removed through catalytic converters or charcoal filters.

The bottom line is, of course, cost. In an exercise carried out by McDonnell Douglas, it was shown that airlines can save 62,000 gallons of fuel a year on each aircraft. However, to bring one C.F.M. of fresh air into the cabin represents an extra 0.012 gallons per hour. If on a 747 flight from New York to Los Angeles with 400 passengers, the ventilation was increased from 10 C.F.M. to 20 C.F.M., the costs would be an extra $240 (0.012 × 10 C.F.M. × 5 hours × 400 = $240). In other words, it is 60 cents per passenger. I am sure that they would be quite willing to pay an extra $1 more on their tickets for cleaner air.

Flying Phenomena

Air travel is like no form of surface transport because its cabin atmosphere is unique. We have already come across unusual factors such as physiological stressors. Here are further examples of conditions and situations that occur.

1. Hyperventilation (Over-breathing). One of the most common conditions that occurs on flights is over-breathing or hyperventilation when passengers are excited or anxious and the cabin is hot and stuffy.

The condition is strange indeed. For not only

17

do the symptoms mimic other illnesses, such as respiratory distress, coronary heart disease, gastro intestinal, central nervous system and thyroid diseases, but they can also cause an insensitivity to pain. This feature is used in voodoo or tribal ceremonies where mutilation is practised.

The gamut of effects include numbness, a tingling in the face or limbs, dizziness, cramps, blurred vision, fatigue, an irritable unproductive cough, fibrositis of different parts of the torso, heartburn, burping, a choking sensation, 'emotional' sweating (palms and armpits), hallucinations, free-floating anxiety and ultimately unconsciousness.

What happens as a result of the rapid shallow breathing, is that excessive amounts of carbondioxide are blown off. Consequently, there is hypocarbia or a low-level of the gas occurring in the blood which in turn alters the acid-alkali balance. The blood becomes more alkaline and inhibits the activity of the enzymes. This affects the cardiovascular and central nervous systems.

Hyperventilation can be stopped through a simple device. Place an airsickness bag over the nose and mouth and breathe into it. Once you rebreathe the expired air for a minute or two, the fast breathing will cease.

Do not try to prevent hyperventilation through breathing oxygen or drinking alcohol. Both these remedies merely aggravate the condition. Like oxygen in the pressurised cabin, there is a similar lack of carbon dioxide on board at the start of each flight. However, because of the inadequate ventilation, there is a gradual increase until the concentrations become excessive.

2. Medication. The effects of drugs on the body may be moderated or increased when you are exposed to the hypoxia and hypocarbia of the pressurised cabin, and the desynchronization of your biological rhythms through time zone changes. Therefore, check with your doctor about reducing or increasing the dosage of your medication before the flight, particularly long-haul.

Epileptics may have to increase the dose because excessive fatigue, excitement of travel and oxygen lack can well provoke an attack. On the other hand, diabetic passengers may have to increase their dose of insulin when travelling west and decrease it when flying east on longhual flights. (This inverse dosage was confirmed recently by Finnish researchers.)

3. Aqualung or Scuba Diving. Arrange to have your last dive at least 12 hours before departure. Otherwise you will suffer from decompression sickness. If you have exceeded a depth of 30 feet wait for at least 24 hours before you depart.

Decompression sickness is a condition that is characterised by severe pain in the muscles and joints, cramp and difficulty in breathing. It is caused by a too rapid return to the surface. However, if you fly too soon after a dive the lower pressure of the cabin produces the same effect.

The pain, I can assure you, is excruciating and one economist I know passed out on board with it. As a result, he now suffers also from aerophobia. The cause of the distress was the rapid release of the nitrogen, which earlier had been absorbed into the body fluids and tissues due to high pressure under water. Bubbles of the gas appear all over in the nervous system, joints, muscles and lungs.

4. Concorde. As the supersonic aircraft flies at 60,000 ft and over, there are greater concentrations of ozone and levels of radiation. Although the aircraft does not offer passengers protection against radiation, it does against the toxic effects of ozone. There is an exception, however, the first three minutes of its descent, when the platinum filter is ineffective due to the drop in temperature. That is the moment to hold a handkerchief over your nose. In some instances, the presence of the gas can provoke an asthma attack.

5. Women. Flying tends to affect female passengers more because of the complex nature of their physiology:

Periods. If you fly on the first day of your period, you may find that it will be heavy. Avoid this if you can. Constant time zone changes will upset your menstrual cycle. If you are a frequent flyer, you may experience irregular periods and/or difficult and painful ones. Some flight attendants have to be grounded for a sufficient time if they want to have children. This enables their menstrual cycle to function normally.

Contraceptive pill. Take the pill the same time every day. This can be achieved in different time zones by having a watch synchronised to your home time. A neater suggestion is to have a wrist-watch with two movements. Another aspect of the pill is that it can increase the risk of blood clots. If you are overweight, over 35 and/or smoke as well, the risk can be doubled.

I.U.D. If you have an intrauterine device it can become displaced during a flight or flights due to gas expansion. Therefore, have it checked by your gynaecologist.

Expectant mothers. Do not fly during the first 12 weeks because of the foetus's sensitivity to radia-tion, and as the incidence of congenital anomalies increases with prolonged hypoxia. Avoid air travel also after the 34–35th week for longhaul, and after the 36th week for shorthaul. The reason for the latter is the fact that the flight environment may induce labour and any complications that arise cannot be dealt with in the cabin. In addition, many health insurance companies do not cover the delivery in any other location than in a hospital.

Before you fly longhaul consult your gynaeco-logist about whether there is a likelihood of a mis-carriage. At the check-in desk, you should ask for an aisle seat in a non-smoking section and near the toilet.

You may also require supplemental oxygen if you have a history of premature labour or suffer from a disorder like toxemia.

On board, drink lots of water, take frequent short walks and do calf muscle exercises to prevent clotting in the leg veins.

Wear the seatbelt around the pelvis.

Avoid gaseous drinks and food that produces gas like beans or curries as the gas expansion internally can cause discomfort.

Avoid scuba diving at all times and high altitude destinations.

If you want to avoid chemical remedies to prevent insect bites, try a skin cream like Avon Skin-So-Soft which is said to have repellant properties against fleas and mosquitos.

Personality. After several years of longhaul flying, flight attendants may experience hormonal changes that can result in hair loss. There also may be changes in the personality. They may become obsessively tidy or clean and develop an obsessive-compulsive neurosis.

6. Children. Children, who have a higher water content than adults and are more sensitive to water loss, should be given small amounts of water at frequent intervals. They are also more at risk from dehydration, particularly when they are suffering from unresolved gastro-enteritis.

To help with pressure changes during the ascent or descent, infants should be offered a dummy or pacifier, and older children, chewing gum or boiled sweets. When they have bad colds or problem ears or teeth, it is best not to travel until they are well.

Newborn infants should not travel before 10–12 days. The air pockets in the lungs may not be fully expanded and the hypoxic atmosphere in the cabin may cause respiratory distress.

7. Inflight Infectious Diseases. People who have contagious diseases, like measles and chickenpox, should not fly. This is extremely important as now more than ever, there is a greater risk of the spread of disease aboard aircraft, due to the increased practice of recycling stale air. It can spread by sneezing, coughing, direct contact or through fabric or paper (fomites).

Tuberculosis may well be contagious under such conditions but there is no evidence that the human immunodeficiency virus (A.I.D.S.) can be transmitted through the air or by casual hand contact. There was also a case of stopover malaria recorded while the doors of an aircraft were open at Abidjan Airport, Ivory Coast, and a passenger was bitten by a mosquito.

If you are overly concerned about the problem, I suggest you may do two things.
1. Wear plastic eye-nose goggles that cover the nose and eyes which are used by hospital staff in children's wards. These will reduce the frequency of catching certain respiratory viruses.
2. Use Daniele Ryman's therapeutic Inflight comfort kits.*

8. A Miscellany of Conditions and Tips.
Wearers of contact lenses should apply lens solution during the flight as these dry out.

Sinusitis sufferers may benefit from using a Daniele Ryman nasal and sinus refresher and/or inhaling the mist from water spray.

Any screw top bottles or jars should be tightened as these may open due to changes in air pressure.

Ears may cause you pain during a descent. This may be relieved through swallowing, chewing gum or trying the Valsalva manoeuvre. The latter consists of inhaling, closing the nose with the thumb and forefinger, and exhaling with the mouth shut. If you have a bad cold use a decongestant spray before you descend.

Skin conditions (eg eczema) can be irritated by

*Available from Daniele Ryman boutique, Park Lane Hotel, Piccadilly, London, W1Y 8BX.

the dryness of the cabin so you should use a compress or water spray on the affected area. Application of a moisturiser or rehydration gel may only aggravate the condition.

If you fly direct to a resort for skiing, mountain trekking or climbing, you may consider taking a diamox (acetazolamide) on arrival as it will help regularize breathing at high altitude.

CHAPTER THREE

THE FEARFUL FLYER

Aerophobia

Flying phobia can be an isolated problem or one of the many fears of agoraphobia. The latter is a fear of open or public spaces that can result in the sufferer becoming housebound.

There are four elements of flying that are particularly feared.
1. The possibility of a crash.
2. The confinement in a closed space such as a cabin.
3. The apparent instability of an aircraft.
4. Heights.

Women passengers tend to present with a flying fear more often than do men. Of the aircrew who suffered from the phobia, it was found that they were more likely to have more marital and sexual problems than those who did not.

The anxiety is generally relieved with the aid of alcohol or sedatives. However, in some passengers it is displaced into sex.

How to Take Out the Fear From Flying

The first step is the acceptance of the fact that we are all afraid of flying. It is an unnatural phenomenon for mankind and had we meant to fly, we would have evolved with wings.

Instead, we have developed with a protective mechanism to prevent us from falling, the Moro reflex. This is a grasping response to any stimulus that suggests falling, which a newborn baby exhibits. In other words, we are all born with an instinctive fear of heights. Therefore, the stigma of being a member of the white knuckle brigade or a coward does not apply. Take a hard-nosed frequent flyer, put him in an aircraft during severe C.A.T. (clear air turbulence) and it is likely that he will emerge a fearful flyer.

Paul Getty, the oilman, never flew again after he had experienced several tornadoes during a flight in 1942. He sent his agent, Claus von Bulow, around the world instead.

Tips on how to deal with the fear of flying follow. As it is different in each of us, choose whichever method or methods that appeal to you.

1. The acceptance that flying is an unnatural activity for human beings. Therefore, it is realistic to experience some sort of fear. This is a healthy reaction.

2. Have a medical examination with an aviation medical specialist to ensure that there is no physiological basis to that fear. For example, people with a mitral valve prolapse tend to complain of anxiety. There is also the case of the dysfunction of the inner ear, which affects the sense of balance and movement of the head. This condition produces symptoms of headache, in-balance, vertigo, nausea and those who suffer from it can develop agoraphobia and anxiety. This aspect is often ignored by psychologists and psychiatrists who rarely have screening programmes for fearful flyers.

3. Check that you are breathing normally on board because faulty breathing can trigger a panic attack. If you find that you are over-breathing, i.e. breathing fast and shallow, you are a step away from effective treatment. The first thing you do is reach for a sick bag and place it over your nose and mouth. Rebreathe your expired air. After a minute or so, your breathlessness will stop and your fear will cease.

To effect a longterm cure, you may have to change your breathing habits from being a fast thoracic (chest) breather to a slow deep diaphragmatic one. Essentially, this means not breathing through your mouth and/or chest but through your nose and stomach. To breathe slowly pause briefly between the in-breath and the out-breath. A consultation with a chest physician or a physiotherapist would be helpful.

There may be additional benefits from deep breathing or breathing from the diaphragm. The psychological advisor to the U.S. Olympic fencing team taught this method to two members, who were having psychological problems before bouts. As a result, their performance and nerves greatly improved. I also know of a top antique dealer, Pamela Howell, who uses this technique to her advantage. When she becomes too excited during negotiations, she excuses herself and retreats to the loo. There she practices diaphragmatic breathing and returns calm and relaxed to close the deal.

4. Bring along magazines or books that you enjoy reading. If you are engrossed in a story or article, time passes quickly and you are unlikely to think about your surroundings. A useful technique to try.

5. Take Teddy with you! It works for the Royal Military Academy, Sandhurst, and can work for you too. There they have an Edward Bear Parachute Club in which their mascot – a teddy bear with a parachute – jumps first from an aircraft. He sets the example to other officer cadets who want to train as parachutists and acts as a drifter – to show the direction of the wind. This remarkable idea was introduced by General Sir Richard Worsley in 1950. It has encouraged many Sandhurst cadets over the years to jump in spite of the adrenalin high and cold sweat. Now you know too why a cuddly toy can help you beat your fear. If it can, you can!

6. Some people bring along a lucky charm or talisman whenever they fly. It puts their mind at

rest and they are less apprehensive on board. One friend of mine always travels with a Montblanc pen. Once she arrived at the airport without it and promptly bought another in the duty-free shop – an expensive purchase but it provides her with peace of mind whenever she flies.

7. Find a sympathetic listener. Talk to a flight attendant or a fellow passenger about your fear. Such a conversation, particularly with a sympathetic flight attendant, goes a long way to reducing your apprehension. Time passes quickly and you can forget that you are on an aircraft.

8. Familiarise yourself with the mechanics of flying. The simplest way to do this is to ask to see the flight deck. There the captain (who sits on the left hand side) and his First Officer will be able to answer any of your questions. The most common one, of course, is how the aircraft stays up there. You may also wish to read entry number 10 which may reassure you and assist you in your understanding of flying.

9. A quick way to get you out of a state of panic on board is to splash your face with cold water. This can be done in the toilet or you may use a water spray on your face several times during a flight. Apply any cold object, eg ice, to parts of your body and the shock can change your attitude. A cold bath or shower or swim before departure could also be a great benefit before your trip.

10. Try to master the mechanics of flying. The simplest way to do this is to ask to see the cockpit. There the captain (who sits in the left hand seat) and his First Officer will be able to answer any of your questions. On the flight deck, the first switches to catch your eye will be the control panel just under the front windshields. Here you can tell what the airspeed is, the altitude above the ground, the aircraft's position, the alignment of the earth's horizon with the artificial horizon and the flight director.

27

Between the two seats are a set of four levers. These are the throttles or thrust levers for the engines. Above the windshields will be the overhead switch panel and on the right the flight engineer's panel. By moving the control column (which looks like a half moon steering wheel of a car) forward or backward, the pilot can force the nose of the aircraft up or down.

The most common question asked is how the plane manages to stay up. It would be better to be framed 'how does a plane fly?' Like a bird for they better have wings. A bird can be described as a living plane for each wing functions as a combined propeller-wing. We have all seen a bird take off – quickly in the case of a small bird and slowly with larger birds like swans or geese. With the latter, there is a cycle of up and down strokes, and it takes some time before it clears the water and is into the air.

On the other hand, a Boeing 747 requires a thrust of 200,000 lbs from its four jet engines, a speed of 180 m.p.h. and a runway distance of 8,500 ft (less if there is a wind) to become airborne. What a performance! Once up in the air, the plane stays there because of the lift it gets from the wings and the power from the engines that propel it.

If any analogy is appropriate, it is the sea and a ship. The sea has waves, currents, tides and whirlpools as does the sky on a much larger scale. The aircraft flies or wings its way across the sky and behaves under you like a ship – a stable and broadbeamed one. The 'control touch' is similar to that of a tiller on a sailboat, and at times requires no steering at all. It flies itself too. Everything in the design balances because of where the centre of gravity is, where the wings are attached and their exact angle and because of the tail fins.

What passengers need to disabuse themselves of is the notion that the air is nothing. You cannot swim unless you believe that water will carry you. The air has mass, substance and power to hold the aircraft up. The best way to test this is in a parachute jump. When you delay opening the parachute and fall free for 500 or 1,000 ft, the air turns out to be something heavy against which you could almost lie as if on a bed. It is not a void.

The airframe of which the aircraft is built is stronger than steel but many times lighter. Not only can it withstand extreme changes in temperature from 120 degrees F in the tropics to 70 degrees F below freezing at high altitude, but various stresses of flying. The landing gear in a 'concrete leveller' or hard landing will be able to withstand three times its loaded weight of 400 tons. There is also the pressurisation stresses to the fuselage and the strength and flexibility of the wings in chopping air which can flap some ten feet or more.

11. Understand the noises associated with the operation of the aircraft. The main door of a 747 thumps as it shuts on the runway, the engines start with a whine, and as each generator is checked by the engineer the lights dim in the cabin.

When the plane taxis towards lift-off position, bouncing on the rough surfaces, the engine noise is louder but not its loudest. On the point of take-off, when it seems to scream, sometimes there is a clatter as loose meal trays in the galley fall. Normal take-off is about 50 seconds and when the flaps come up, the aircraft sinks slightly. As it climbs there will be a sudden hush as the engines are throttled back for the noise-abatement procedure.

At the top of the climb (T.O.C.), there will be a further reduction in engine noise. You will hear a low hum from now on throughout the cruise. To set a proper course, the aircraft banks by up to 25 degrees. About 100 miles from the destination, the descent begins and the engines become quieter. Through a window you may be able to see the flaps moving into place as they slow the aircraft and hear the whine of the hydraulic engine. The loudest noise occurs when the undercarriage is lowered. Just above the ground there is a hush, which is followed by a crash and a jolt as the main wheels connect. The nose wheels drop and as the engines reverse, there is a shuddering howling noise. This is the moment to applaud. The worst is over.

12. Drugs and booze are bad news. Beware of tranquillisers or beta-blockers and alcohol as the pressurised cabin increases their potency. If they are mixed, ie tranquillizers and alcohol, it can cause memory loss at your destination. I know the beta-blockers relieve the symptoms of dizziness, breathlessness and sweating, and are non-addictive. But my view is that to resort to either or both is no remedy. At best they will deal with the symptoms and not the cause. Rather, tackle the contents of your thoughts.

13. Another way of building your confidence is to prepare for the worst. Here is advice on how to survive a crash.

The survival rate worldwide of passengers in a crash has risen in the past two decades from 33% to 60%. Although the chance of being involved in a crash is about one in a million, there are various recommendations that might just save a life.

There are two main aspects of a crash – the impact and the fire together with an explosion and/or smoke. If you survive the first get ready for the next. As a rule of thumb you have between 30–60 seconds to get out. At the first sign of any trouble go into a 'crash brace' position. This means that you place your head in your lap and cover it with your hands and elbows. A backward facing seat in such a situation would be far safer.

General tips to be heeded before your next trip, ie be prepared:

1. Book a seat in a row at the exit, preferably the overwing exit, or near one. An aisle seat is a better choice than a window seat.

2. Go on an air-crash survival course, eg the Stark Survival Company, Banana City, Florida, U.S.A. There you may learn that exit windows

are heavy, weighing over 50 lbs. It is not easy to lift one out and instructions to unlatch it may be obscured by thick smoke.

3. Buy a smoke hood. This is a transparent mask which filters out smoke, enabling the passenger to breathe for about 30 minutes during an evacuation and folds into a small pouch. It is available from Survival Products in the U.S. at 0101 (817) 923-0300.

4. Avoid polyster and nylon clothing as these fabrics are highly inflammable, and ensure that the clothing covers most of your body. T-shirts and shorts should not be worn. High heel shoes may puncture a life raft or emergency slide. Carry an extra pair of spectacles/eyeglasses or use a safety strap.

5. Memorise the exits on each flight and count how many rows there are between them and your seat.

6. If you travel with infants under two years old, who qualify for free travel, buy them tickets and place them in child-restraint seats. Consult the F.A.A.'s 'Child/Infant Safety Seats, Recommended for Use in Aircraft', tel: 0101 (202) 267 3479 or at Community and Consumer Liaison Division, APA-200, 800 Independence Ave., S.W. Washington D.C., 20591. Children can easily be thrown about during a crash landing.

Specific tips for a fast exit from a smoke-filled and burning aircraft:

1. While you move towards the exit or opening in the fuselage, keep your head low to avoid smoke or toxic fumes. If you have a smoke hood, it makes your progress easier.

2. Do not crawl on the floor as you could be trampled by others in the scramble to evacuate.

3. Look for emergency lights on the floor which change colour at the seat rows next to the exit doors.

4. At the exit check for any hazard outside before leaving the plane.

5. Should the escape route be an evacuation slide, jump, legs together and feet first, into the middle with arms across your chest. If the slide has failed to inflate, climb down it instead.

6. Should the escape route be an overwing exit, throw the door out of the plane so as not to block the passage. Look for a marked walkway highlighted in non-slip paint. If the wing flaps are extended slide down them on your back, feet first with hands at your side. If not, jump down.

7. On the ground, move as fast as you can away from the plane in case of an explosion. The best direction is against the wind to avoid the smoke or toxic fuel.

I must confess it is quite salutary to be familiar with this safety drill, because I for one feel more confident about a crash. I at least have some idea of what I am up against.

14. Some passengers opt for an instinctive solution. They join the Mile High Club. Such a response could be called inverse sublimation. But nowadays, it is termed displacement. Out of two experiences, aerophobia and sex, there are people who feel that the latter is more socially acceptable. This substitution is known as compensatory displacement.

15. If you have got as far as this and still feel inadequate about overcoming your fear of flying, then you have two further options. Take a course and/or read a book based on such a course. In the

U.K., British Airways run Nervous Flyers courses that cost over £100, telephone: 061 832 7972. A cheaper alternative is to read the book, *Taking the Fear Out of Flying* by Maurice Yaffe (David & Charles) at £5.95 a copy.

In the U.S., the oldest course is by Captain T.W. Cummings, 0101 (305) 261 7042, and expect to pay £300. His book, *Freedom From Fear of Flying* (Pocket Books) sells at £3.95 (I.S.B.N. – 0671 628 631) and the audio cassette with a booklet, £25.

In Germany, Lufthansa has Relaxed Flying courses at eight airports. Contact Barbara Fose in Frankfurt or Silvia Texter in Munich, telephone: 069 696 8757 or 089 391 739 respectively. For other countries, the best place to check for courses or books are the national airlines. There are also treatments such as desensitization – a form of relaxation, which is favoured by the R.A.F. Institute of Aviation Medicine, and cognitive behaviour. In the U.S., this can be provided by a cognitive behavioural therapist or a behaviour therapist. In the U.K., the equivalent would be a chartered clinical psychologist. Elaine Forman in London (telephone: 081 459 3428) is a psychologist who undertakes such treatments.

CHAPTER FOUR

HOW TO OVERCOME JETLAG

Jetlag is the most common complaint to afflict frequent flyers on longhaul trips. As time and money is lost because of the physical and mental impairments of the condition, all sorts of remedies are tried without much success.

However, the intrinsic weakness of these remedies is that none take into account the effects of the flight environment. This is what I have done with the Airwise Method. Most frequent flyers will find that it coincides with what they have been doing instinctively anyway. I have merely provided the rationale and refined the technique to make it more effective.

On July 20, 1991, I flew halfway across the world from London, crossed 12 time zones and arrived in Auckland. I spent three days in the city before flying to Sydney, Melbourne, Los Angeles and was back in London within 10 days. For me it was an historic trip, because I never suffered from jetlag, both on the outward-bound and inward journeys.

Jetlag is a Misnomer

For some time now I have been having second thoughts about the so-called medical condition of jetlag. What I mean is whether it exists or not. As it stands, it is defined as dysrhythmia or desynchronosis, which basically represents the disruption of your biological rhythms. But can this really be a disease or illness?

I know it also involves crossing time zones, with the resultant lengthening or shortening of days, and a whole host of symptoms. These I will not bother to mention as they are familiar to all flyers.

34

The seeds of doubt were sown by four N.A.S.A. scientists (Winget, Deroshia, Markley and Holley) while I was working on my first book, *The Curse of Icarus*. They had written a review of the condition for the journal, *Aviation, Space and Environmental Medicine*, and had mentioned a similarity of the symptoms with shift work. I was furious at the time. How could they compare such a mundane and menial task with an aerospace activity?

There were so many other factors in the flight environment that such a comparison was meaningless. At its extreme, shiftwork involved a change from working during the day to working at night or vice versa. When that occurred you may lose several nights of sleep before you settled into a routine. In some cases, shiftwork was more disruptive because people had to alternate between a week of work during the day, and a week during the night.

In the air, you not only had to deal with changes to your biological rhythms, but also culture shock. You shot from one part of the globe to another and faced a new climate, foreign language, unfamiliar surroundings, different people and strange customs.

But I think the main objection was one of status. Shiftworkers in the main are people who work on production lines in factories or nurses in hospitals. Their status is generally considered low compared with frequent flyers or jetsetters, who have money, position and power.

There is another aspect too. To write about jetlag imparts a certain amount of glamour to the writer, for travel equals excitement and fascination with other cultures. Even the medical author is seduced by the terminology: synchronizers (zeitgebers), circadian rhythms, transmeridian, multiple time zone changes, sleep-awake oscillators, disoreintation etc.

The remedies also have their attraction. They vary from bright lights that reset the circadian pacemaker, feast and fast diets, hormone pills that have yet to be marketed, aromatherapy 'Awake'

35

and 'Asleep' fragrances, sleep credits and deficits and short-acting hypnotics that cause amnesia if mixed with alcohol. Any day now I am expecting an 'Alice in Wonderland' antidote, a magic potion, which will lengthen or shorten our inner day to fit in with the new time zones.

I now think the whole thing is a sham. Had jetlag been a true medical disease like measles, they would have long ago come up with an antidote or vaccine to cure it.

No, jetlag is a misnomer. It is not an illness but another word for fatigue – unrelievable fatigue. It was coined by John Foster Dulles, a U.S. Secretary of State, who blamed his irascibility and poor judgement, that led to the Suez Crisis in 1956, on the multiple time zones he had crossed. This was the period when the Comet and Boeing 707 was just being introduced.

Since then, it has become a byword for unmitigated fatigue in jetsetters of all professions. But because of the glamour of travel, jetlag is also a symbol of international status. It is the latter which has blurred the issue. No one will give up such status without a fight.

If one could prove that jetlag was nothing more than extreme exhaustion, people would be loath to believe it as they do of M.E., an obscure disease with similar symptoms. If one went on further and demonstrated that this was a result of your own self-indulgence – overeating and drinking – they would believe it even less.

However, like scientists or medical researchers, I have experimented on myself on several occasions. Fortunately, the experiment is simple and can be tried by any passenger.

I conducted the experiment on three occasions that involved 2×24 hour, 2×36 hour and 2×11 hour flights. These were two return trips to New Zealand along the Western and Eastern routes, and a return flight to Los Angeles respectively.

First, I defined the problem. The body is at rest or sedentary for most of the trip and as a result requires minimal amounts of calories. Yet the intake of food and alcoholic drink is excessive. On the other hand, the cabin environment creates a shortage of oxygen and moisture in the body. So the metabolism is thrown into a conflict. It is pushed to digest the food and drink, and convert them into energy, while being deprived of the vital ingredients of water and oxygen.

What I did was to go with the flow. 1. I cut down on the food and drink as best as I could. 2. I kept myself well watered on board and oxygenated on the ground during transit stops. That was my method.

The first opportunity I had to try my experiment was on a trip to New Zealand on July 20, 1991. This is the longest route in the world and I would spend 24 hours in the air. I flew on an Air New Zealand flight: a Boeing 747-400, whose route was London to Auckland via Los Angeles. Take-off time was 1700 hours. From London to L.A. I refused the two meals offered and drank one glass of still bottled water every hour. When we landed in L.A., 11 hours later, I spent most of the two hours on the ground constantly walking in the transit lounge. I only sat down once and on that occasion, I ate a large orange.

On the second leg of the trip, I again passed up the two meals and drank my quota of water. I relaxed and slept for several hours. One of the things that kept me abstemious was the thought of having breakfast on arrival which was scheduled at 6am. I had followed my experiment so well that when I arrived at my hotel I was starving! I felt a kinship with the great flyer, Lindbergh, who had only eaten one sandwich during the 34 hours it had taken him to fly the Atlantic in 1927.

The Results

Fortunately, I was booked into the Pan Pacific Hotel's Club Pacific, which comprises the top four floors, and has a lounge with a panoramic view of Auckland. A sight appropriate enough for my triumph, I told myself. There I indulged myself in an English breakfast, which is served from 7am. However, as I still had a reserve of willpower, I skipped the lamb chops and the hominy grits. But the freshly fried egg was the best I had tasted in years!

One factor I had not accounted for was the psychological. I felt terrific. And over the next four days as I was free of jetlag, this feeling of exhilaration would increase. After breakfast, I read the New Zealand Herald and rang some friends. Then I went for a three-hour stroll around central Auckland, a city I had never been to before.

My friends, upon hearing how good I felt, took me to a party that evening – partly, I felt, to see me sag with jetlag. But I stayed the course and went to bed at 1am. I slept well. Although I woke up at 6am for a short period, I went back to sleep until 9am. For the next five nights, my sleep pattern did not alter. But the fact that I felt I had overcome jetlag put me in a positive mental state. It was most unfortunate for my friends, because at any pretext I was liable to tell them how good I was feeling.

Since I was on a promotional tour, I was on the move again across the Tasman – only a three-hour flight to Sydney, and then to Melbourne. My next big hop would be on the Sunday when I would return to Auckland for a night flight to Los Angeles. The travelling time was 11 hours 55 minutes and two meals were included – supper and breakfast again. I stuck to my spartan diet of water and more water. The total flying time was 14 hrs 55 minutes from Melbourne to Los Angeles.

After checking into the Beverly Wiltshire at about 6pm the same day, I went for a two-hour walk around Beverly Hills. By the time my lungs were well ventilated, my circulation system oxygenated, I was rather hungry. For the next few days I did not exhibit any of the usual symptoms of jetlag except for waking on two nights at irregular hours, but immediately going back to sleep again.

Four days later, I took the evening flight back to London with a flying time of 10 hours 25 minutes.

But before I stepped on board I had a half-hour swim in the hotel pool, and a glass of champagne in the Air New Zealand V.I.P. lounge. On this flight, I was brave enough to sample some hors d'oeuvres with my water, but to the chagrin of the First Class flight attendant, skipped the dinner and breakfast. Ensuring that I was well watered at all times, even drinking 3–4 cups before I slept, I arrived in good shape. Thereafter, with the exception of the odd night of waking suddenly but going back to sleep immediately, I was free of jetlag and its symptoms.

Further Experiments

Within the next six months, I had two further opportunities to try my airwise method. The first was a return trip on a charter to New Zealand on November 28, 1991, via Sharjah, Singapore and Cairns which took 36 hours. There were two differences in my experiment and one variation in my method. I travelled in Economy Class with a companion who later complained that I had starved her. Instead of eating an orange at the transit stops of Sharjah and Singapore, I varied this with kiwifruit. Lengthy walks at the three transit stops were still undertaken.

Again, the short sleep disruption was noted in both of us, but we had little trouble in falling asleep soon after. On our return to London we stuck to the airwise method. I must admit I did not look forward to this horrendous trip, and have since admired Kiwis who think nothing of crossing the line on O.E. (Overseas Experience) to and from Europe.

In May, 1992, my companion (now my wife) and I flew non-stop to Los Angeles on a Virgin Atlantic flight 007. We were in Upper Class and although I was prepared to undertake the airwise method, she was not except for drinking water. The lunch menu was too tempting for her – they had courses by Raymond Blanc – and a New Zealand Sauvignon Blanc. So she ate lightly and had a glass of wine. When the afternoon tea arrived, she did the same. I maintained my spartan attitude throughout. But I indulged in another way by breathing 100% oxygen from a portable canister for one and a half hours towards the end of the flight. My head felt clear after this, and I never had a headache which I sometimes get on board (see Hypoxia on page 5).

On arrival in Los Angeles, my hunger was on cue. My reactions were similar to my other trips. But my fiance felt irritable for three days – perhaps the price for indulging in the cuisine on board.

After a week, we returned to London. On the inward-bound Virgin flight, my fiance ate lightly during lunch, drank a glass of wine and had a slice of walnut and cherry cake with tea. She also downed copious glasses of water. I being my spartan self, stuck to water alone.

Back home in Oxford, we both experienced the usual sleep disturbances, and on one occasion, my fiance could not go back to sleep. She was also irritable for a couple of days. The consumption of food and drink on board could have been responsible for the irritability. I, on the other hand, generally felt good and free of jetlag.

Not bad, I thought – I have finally licked jetlag. The relief I felt was incredible, and the exhilaration. What should not be underestimated is the psychological boost you get when you are successful.

Summary of Airwise Method

Before I summarise the method I have used, I will anticipate a question that many frequent flyers or pilots will ask. How did I manage to sleep? Did I use sleeping pills? I will answer the second question first – no, I did not take any drugs to sleep.

On arrival, I would try to fit in immediately with the local time. If it was night or day I would stay up until 2200–2300 hours. On the other hand, if I felt like a sleep during the day I would do so for the maximum of an hour. To sleep longer would badly disrupt my sleeping pattern. But the first thing I would do was to have a meal, with or without alcohol. This would be followed by exercise; either a walk or a swim. Later, when I went to bed, I would rub some 'Asleep'* fragrance around my nasal area. The familiar relaxing aromas are enough to send me off to sleep.

My method, which for want of a better name, can be called the Airwise Method. It essentially consists of counter-acting the negative effects of the flight environment. Excess and lack (E.A.L.) are the dominant features. The oxygen lack of between 20–26% can be remedied on board by conserving oxygen:

1. If you sleep or lie at rest you consume 0.24 litres/min compared with 0.34 litres/min when you sit and rest, or 0.85 litres/min when you walk.

2. The intestine region of your body accounts for about 25% of the total oxygen consumption. In addition, the secretion of stressor hormones also slows down digestion. So it is best to limit the intake of food that will require extra oxygen to digest it. On the ground at transit stops, you can easily oxygenate your body through exercise.

The other lack you have to correct is water. The relative humidity in the cabin can drop to about 3% which is eight times less than the R.H. in a centrally heated room. The body needs on average 2½ litres of water per day to carry out its functions. Therefore, you must drink more water on board.

The excess referred to is, of course, the food and drink available on the aircraft. This should be avoided as it not only decreases the oxygen lack further through digestion. Consumption of alcohol and diuretics like tea and coffee also increase the dehydration. Then there is the excess of gas, which expands to 35% and plays a minor role. What conclusions can one draw from my self-experiment?

*Available from Daniele Ryman boutique, Park Lane Hotel, Piccadilly, London W1Y 8BX.

Conclusion

1. The flight environment is usually ignored in any jetlag literature or tests, yet as has been demonstrated, it is a significant element.
2. If you can come to terms with this environment, you have little else to deal with other than a small degree of disturbed sleep. In fact, the changes experienced are less disruptive than for people on continual shiftwork.
3. In view of the two points already mentioned, can jetlag be dignified by the name of disease or medical condition? I think not.

The Airwise Method

This is a simple, radical and effective remedy. It requires resolve and the greater the resolve, the bigger the success. As a result, there are variations on the method. Essentially, it requires your body to be in a state of semi-hibernation to lessen the combined stresses of oxygen deprivation, dehydration, slower circulation and gas expansion.

1. Rest, relax or sleep. This ensures that you use as little oxygen as possible where there can be a deficit in pressure of up to 26%. As the brain is the most sensitive of all the organs in the body to such a deficit, your mental efficiency is affected. Therefore, do not expect to do any serious work on board but rather read something light or watch a comedy. Avoid thrillers or the news as these can release stressor hormones in your body. Best of all – sleep.

2. Drink water as if there were no tomorrow. Even consume a couple of glasses before you go to sleep. For convenience, if you are in Economy Class, take along your own supply of still mineral water (1.5 or 2 litres).

3. Eat nothing! Such an attitude requires a willpower, particularly if you are in the first class with its impeccable cuisine, and the senior flight attendant treats your resolve with disdain.

The answer, of course, is to ask for a doggy bag. I once saw a Japanese woman doing just that on a Dublin to London flight, after she had asked her husband's permission.

For the abstemious, take along an orange or two, or settle for a green salad if you can get one. But such a fast is not as bad as it seems, because your stomach will be filled with a lake of water anyway. The additional benefit is that you will expend little or no energy on digestion.

4. Avoid alcohol or tea and coffee. These are counter-productive to drinking water, as they both cause you to pass more fluid. If you must drink alcohol, have wine rather than spirits, which have a higher alcohol content, and limit yourself to one glass before take-off. It is worth nothing that red wine is less diuretic than white and steer clear of beer because of the high gas content (see The balloon body, page 6).

5. At stopovers, exercise as much as possible. In the transit lounge, I walk nonstop at a leisurely pace. If I sit down at all, it is to eat an orange. As the body has been deprived of oxygen, it is important to fill the lungs and oxygenate the blood as fast as possible. (Jogging would be a far more efficient way of achieving this but I know of no transit lounge where this is possible). At the same time, the exercise enables you to relax or sleep more easily later on board.

Success. On arrival, nothing will match the exhilaration of your triumph over jetlag. A rare feat indeed until more passengers become airwise! While you are still travelling, as an inducement to the Airwise Method, you may even think of an appropriate treat to celebrate the event. Throughout my New Zealand trip the thought of having a good English breakfast after arrival was enough for me. The fact that I could have it soon after I had checked into my hotel, made it more pleasurable.

Unconventional methods of avoidance and treatment

Some people believe that these methods work. However, I have only tried the fragrances as a supplement to the airwise method and found them helpful.

1. 'Awake' and 'Asleep' fragrances. Formulated by a leading authority on aromatherapy, Daniele Ryman, these fragrances should be used in your bath or shower on arrival. This method has been around for several years and is used by Air New Zealand, among other airlines. It has achieved an effectiveness rate of 73% in double blind tests involving 300 longhaul cabin crew.

2. Fast and feast diet. Dr C.E. Ehret's programme involves alternate days of light and heavy meals, which is started four days before departure. It is complicated and I have not tried it simply for that reason. Also if you have to cancel your flight or it is delayed, all the effort has been in vain.

CHAPTER FIVE

IMMUNIZATION OF TRAVELLERS

There are certain destinations where immunization or vaccination certificates are compulsory.
Travel agents and embassy officials usually advise
passengers of the particular requirements.

The best way to deal with this, if you have time,
is to ring up your G.P. or physician who will advise
you where you should go. Note that a full
immunization schedule can take two months or
more to accomplish, but valuable protection can
still be gained in less time.

In the U.K. there is also the Department of Health
and Social Services (addresses available in the
appendix), and in the U.S., the Department of
Health in different states or Center of Disease
Control, Atlanta, Georgia 30373, tel: 0101 (404)
639 3311.

If you have a rushed schedule, go directly to an
immunization clinic like British Airways (071 831
5333) or Masta (071 631 4408), where it can be
done immediately. In the U.S. it is preferable to
check with the airline as the list of clinics is too
long to publish. However, you should check
whether any outbreaks of disease have occurred
before you fly and immunization centres can
provide you with up-to-date information.

With regards to the non-compulsory requirements, you may wish to err on the cautious side
and get your jabs for all countries outside northern
Europe, the U.S.A., Canada, New Zealand and
Australia. For example, you could have protection
against typhoid, tetanus, polio, hepatitis A and
yellow fever for Africa and South America. In Asia,
you could have the same immunization programme except for yellow fever. Nowadays, there

are vaccines for most diseases including Hepatitis A.

It is worth noting that with the latter, the vaccination certificate remains valid for ten years but becomes effective only ten days after injection.

Infectious or Contagious Diseases

Besides specific preventive measures, such as immunization, there is also the use of drugs and hints on eating in foreign countries.

The main use of drugs is against malaria, which is considered to be the most dangerous infectious disease of the tropics, and to a certain extent, against diarrhoeal disease. The taking of anti-malarial tablets may be helpful but they are not infallible. Therefore, it is important to apply insect repellant eg deet (diethyl toluamide), Avon Skin-So-Soft or citronella oil, into the skin twice daily and use mosquito nets impregnated with per-methrin over the bed at night. With diarrhoea, there are antidiarrhoeal and antibiotic agents that can be taken. But as this sickness is usually self-limiting – it runs its course after 1–3 days – the agents are not essential.

For the rest it is a question of practising food hygiene. Ensure that you eat food that has just been cooked and thoroughly cooked. It is counter-productive to ask for rare steak as the meat has not been heat sterilised.

If this is not possible eat food from cans or sealed packs. For dessert, choose fruit that you can peel or cut open yourself eg bananas, pineapple, melons, oranges or apples.

On the other hand, having a meal in a luxury hotel or restaurant is no guarantee of cleanliness. I once had a chicken dish in a five-star hotel in Cairo and suffered from a severe bout of diarrhoea. Avoid the following at all costs:

1. Shellfish and prawns because of contaminated seawater.
2. Salads and uncooked vegetables because of the use of nightsoil (human faeces) as fertilizer.

3. Milk and milk products such as icecream and yoghurt, particularly if it is unpasteurized or un-boiled.
4. Ice and untreated or unboiled water. If you cannot get bottled water, disinfect water with iodine or chlorine-based tablets.
5. Food that flies have settled on because of the dangers of faecal-oral transmission of disease.
6. Reheated or cold food which has been left standing in the open.

If you feel you have caught an infectious disease, contact the following soon after arrival:
U.K.: Department of Communicable and Tropical Diseases, East Birmingham Hospital, Bordesley Green Rd., Birmingham B9 5ST. Tel: 021 772 4311.
U.S.: Public Health Service, Division of Quarantine Centers for Disease Control, Atlanta, Georgia 30333. Tel: (call collect) 0101 404 639 1437 or nights, Sunday and holidays 404 639 2888.

A.I.D.S.

The best precaution you can take against H.I.V. when you travel abroad, particularly in out-of-the-way places, is to carry your own sterile medical kit with you. This will ensure that you will reduce the risk of a doctor using contaminated equipment on you – in case of an emergency.

The Medical Advisory Service for Travellers Abroad (M.A.S.T.A.) recommends a kit of hypodermic needles, syringes, swabs and sutures at £13.50. These are available by mail order: 071 631 4408.

Immune System

Frequent air travel appears to lower the resistance to infections. Flight attendants tend to be susceptible to continual colds, chest infections, chronic throat infections and thrush.

Dr David Shlim, Director of C.I.W.E.C. Clinic, Kathmandu, Nepal, has noticed that travellers have a high complication rate for common colds and are more prone to staphylococcal skin infections among other things. As a result of studying them over the past six years, he concluded that they may have a mild reduction in their immune response for unknown reasons.

No Immunization in India

A friend of mine has always had a bad reaction to vaccinations. On a recent trip to India she decided to forgo any protection. Although India, because of all its poverty, disease and reputation for being filthy, is the destination that westerners would think twice about going to, no actual vaccination certificates are required.

However, it is advised that you protect yourself against cholera, typhoid, polio and hepatitis. What she did throughout her four-week stay was to suck three cloves a day and rub her hands and feet (mainly under the soles as they were exposed in sandles) with tea tree oil twice a day.

Her reason for using cloves is that it is a powerful antiseptic, particularly against intestinal parasites, and in the prevention of viral infections. It is also known to boost the immune system. The tea tree oil is an excellent bacteriacide (similar to an antibiotic) and complements the clove.

Although she ate sometimes at roadside stalls – picking out the food on top and in contact with the plate – not out of choice but because there was no other food, she never suffered from any illness. Her companion, a nurse who had completed a full immunization programme, was affected by diarrhoea.

CHAPTER SIX

AIRPORT ENVIRONMENT

Airport

One airport is very much like any other airport and the only difference is the degree of stress found in each. But studies have shown that in such a stressful environment, you cannot build up a resistance to crowdedness, in spite of repeated exposure.

The mere sight of all those people, the high levels of noise and the queues everywhere is enough to trigger the release of stressor hormones such as adrenalin. These natural secretions are the body's response to fear. They raise your blood pressure and speed up your system to the extent that you do things you did not intend to do. For example, you easily become irritable or angry and, to the delight of the airport authorities, make distressed purchases in the duty-free shops.

As the situation is unlikely to change, it is important for you to be an oasis of calm in the stressful airport environment. Arrive early and sit in an airline lounge, in a chapel or a quiet corner to catch up with your reading, work or just yourself. If a shower or swimming pool is available use them as water is the best relaxant before flying. It is better for your health to step on board relaxed than to be anxious, mentally and physically stressed and to be suffering from hypertension. For there are further demands to be made on your body later. Elderly, unfit passengers or mothers with small children should all make use of the electric courtesy carts to take them from check-in to the gates.

I once asked the most senior captain in T.W.A., who had spent three years aloft, what he did at airports on commuter flights. 'I've learnt patience

– the art of killing time gracefully,' he said. 'I always take along a shoulder bag full of things I want to check or read which I hate to spend time on at home.'

Whenever I fly I arrive early and have a glass of champagne an hour before take-off. I find it not only relaxes me but induces a feeling of elation. After all, it is an 'euphorisant' or euphoric. Crowds, stress and delays, and whatever else the airport throws at you can be dismissed with equanimity.

Airline Club Lounge

If your ticket does not entitle you to use an airline lounge, it is a good idea to join an airline club even though you may travel only a couple of times a year. Whatever the cost, the bonus to your health alone is worth the investment. The tranquil surroundings reduce the secretion of stressor hormones in your blood and go a long way to preparing you for a better flight.

Here too you can conduct that final business meeting with greater self-assurance and success than you would if you were in an anxious state, afraid of missing your flight. This is far better than running like the clappers in the airport concourse to catch your plane and one day that exertion could be too much for your heart.

In addition, there are several advantages: comfortable seating and a desk if you want to work; business facilities like telephones, faxes and photocopiers; complimentary beverages and snacks to which you can treat yourself; toilets and restrooms where you can change into more comfortable clothes; and for entertainment – magazines, newspapers and a television.

The receptionist will also inform you when your flight is ready for boarding and some times take you to the gate. I remember on two occasions, when I had to gird my loins for the return trip, Auckland to London, and how the two hours in the Air New Zealand lounge were most beneficial. The unpleasant prospect of spending the next 24 hours in the air disappeared in that room with its beautiful view of the sparkling Manukau Harbour.

Pacemakers and Body Bullets

If you are fitted with a pacemaker inform the security staff of the fact before you pass through the metal detector. In the U.K., U.S. and most western countries, the magnetic field is at a level that will not induce changes in the electrical components of pacemakers. However, this may not be the case in other countries and as a result, it can interfere with your instrument's rhythms.

Be safe and sure and tell the staff who will instead give you a personal body check. If you travel frequently, I have heard that you can apply for an international medical certificate that states you have a pacemaker.

The same advice applies to passengers with bits of metal in their bodies as a result of operations or old bullets from war wounds. There was an old soldier at Hong Kong Airport who caused himself a lot of trouble because of an old war wound. The Chinese security staff were unsatisfied when they could not find anything on him and yet the metal pinged whenever he went through the detector. It was only once he had stripped down to his underwear that they spotted the scars on his leg and understood. The bullet in his leg caused the problem. A medical certificate would have been a smart solution.

CHAPTER SEVEN

FOOD, DRINK AND ADVICE

It is best to eat before you fly, particularly if it is a night flight, so that you can go to sleep soon after you board. The main reason is that the flight environment is not conducive to digestion or to taste.

Our digestion is sluggish due to oxygen lack and the distension of the alimentary canal because of gas expansion. In addition, any stress on the ground before boarding tends also to slow down digestion.

Airline food, as we know, is another version of fast food because it is precooked or partially cooked before the flight and reheated several hours later on board. Eating haute cuisine in the air is an illusion in spite of the food being prepared by famous chefs. The process is further complicated by the fact that our taste buds are blunted by the atmosphere so we cannot appreciate the finer distinctions of dishes even if they were freshly cooked in the aircraft kitchen. Our noses tend to become congested through the dehydration and are affected by the cool, stale air that is circulated.

There are foods that are gas-forming and add to the swollen cavities of our bodies in flight. These are raw apples, dried beans and peas, cabbage, cauliflower, cucumber, turnips, brussel sprouts and those with a high roughage content. Carbonated drinks and curries fit into the category too.

The only food I would recommend is salad or fruit. If you cannot resist the food put in front of you, pick at it. And should you eat because of boredom, take along anything that interests you such as a game, crossword or book. There are all kinds of fruit to choose from, ie apples, oranges, bananas, peaches, kiwifruit, plums etc. Oranges are good because they contain potassium which we lose on board because of our inactivity; apples contain pectin which is considered useful for the immune system; and bananas contain complex sugars for instant energy. Avoid pears because they have a diuretic effect.

Water

Drink water as if there were no tomorrow when you fly. The air which is drawn off at altitude is drier than any desert on earth. Within an hour of take-off a flower wilts and sliced bread turns stale. That is what happens to your insides!

You have to keep yourself well watered throughout a flight, particularly longhaul. Drink at least a cup of water per hour. If you go to sleep, see that you have 2–3 cups beforehand. The best water to drink is flat and not gaseous as the latter expands in your stomach at altitude.

Juices are no substitute for water. In fact, they could be counter-productive, particularly if they are sweet, because some of the water will have to be used to help the body absorb the sugar. The body will have to retain some water in the intestines to assist this process. Go for bottled water and if you are in Economy Class, it is better to bring your own 2 litre bottle on board.

Alcohol, on the other hand, should be avoided because of its diuretic properties and the fact that the flight environment increases its potency. The most potent alcoholic drinks are spirits such as whisky and brandy which should not be drunk undiluted. A friend who enjoys his booze on board always has water as a chaser after each glass. Another suitable method is to have alcohol with your meal, particularly a glass of red wine if a good vintage is available. Beer has its disadvantage because its fizziness introduces gas into your gut which expands during the flight. With wine, it is better to go for a red rather than a white which has greater diuretic properties.

Airwise Advice

Goose-down

Some passengers find it difficult to sleep on board particularly if they are tall and have to squeeze into the narrow economy seats. However, Angela Baker hit upon the perfect solution. She takes along a goose-down pillow that is easily compressed into her hand luggage.

Upgrade or downgrade gear

A businessman who frequently travels on Concorde never wears a pinstripe on the plane. His usual attire is a blazer and a pair of flannels. However, once on board he changes into something casual: a Champion tracksuit or a sweat shirt and a tracksuit bottom.

A well-travelled publisher, however, recommends always wearing a casual unstructured suit because:

a. Officials are more polite to be-suited passengers.

b. If the airline has to 'bump' people up a class on overcrowded flights they are more likely to select be-suited passengers.

c. If the airline loses his luggage then he does not have to mope around at the hotel and the book fair in a funny track suit.

d. Suits have lots of pockets for wallets, tickets, passports etc.

e. Cab drivers are more likely to stop for a suit.

f. Even a crumpled suit elicits more respect than any other sort of clothing.

Visas

It is essential to check on whether the country to which you are going requires a visa or not. Otherwise, you will be caught short as I was once. On a business trip to the Antipodes, I did not realise that New Zealand and Australia had different regulations for British passport holders. The former did not require a visa while the latter did. My departure from Auckland to Sydney was delayed because the Australian authorities did not allow an airline to carry a passenger without a visa. If they did the airline would be fined $10,000.

Midnight Express, Cairo

Next time you think of stopping off at a destination en route, think twice. A couple of travellers went to Kenya and on the way home decided to visit Egypt. As they stood in the passport control queue at Cairo Airport two burly men asked them if they had a yellow fever certificate. When they admitted that they each did not have one, they were put into a small room and guarded by a soldier with a machine gun.

After being kept there for 24 hours, they were allowed to telephone their consul. They explained that they had been given a choice and asked his advice: either they could take the next plane home or be placed in quarantine for ten days. The latter was a euphemism for being held in jail.

The official was laconic. 'Have you seen Midnight Express?' he asked them. That settled the matter and the travellers decided to leave. Thereafter they were escorted by armed guards to the boarding lounge and later onto the plane. Their fellow passengers gave them a wide berth as they thought they were terrorists or criminals.

Stay Cool

There are two lessons to be learnt whenever you travel. The first is to be unflappable and the second to always have a contingency plan. Many passengers are bumped from aircraft, some in spite of having Business Class tickets which they believed would ensure against such action. You not only have to accept the unpredictability of air travel but not be stressed by it. In the long-term stressor hormones, such as adrenalin, can alter your metabolism. It can cause cardiac arrhythmias, give you trouble with your sleep and generally make you more edgy. Therefore, always have a contingency plan as it is the ideal way to take pressure off you in the case of a delayed flight or a cancellation. Ring your secretary to re-schedule meetings.

There are two strategies to be adopted when you fly. Ensure that you leave your presentation documents as well as clean underwear and a shirt in your hand luggage. This covers you against any loss of baggage in the hold. The other device is to think of alternative routes. Sometimes you can arrive back earlier by taking an alternative route.

Hot Baths

There are a few frequent flyers who do not suffer from jetlag. Archie Clowes, a banker and stockbroker, is one of them. For the past 20 years, he has flown the trans-Atlantic route and believes that jetlag is the result of a hangover. He never drinks on board, except for an occasional glass of wine, and neither does he eat. Whenever he flies, either east or west, he takes a night flight and on arrival has a hot bath. Then he has a nap and is at work or in the office soon after.

CHAPTER EIGHT:

HIGH RISK CONDITIONS

As a result of the physiological stressors of flying, in particular the oxygen deficiency, some diseases can be tipped into a critical phase during or after a flight.

There are guidelines on diseases that can be potentiated:
If the condition interferes with:
1. the lungs' function
2. the heart's function
3. the flow of blood through the circulatory system
4. the oxygen content of the blood
5. or causes the blood to clot easily.

In addition, where there are open sores, ulcers, cysts or inflammation in cavities or semi-cavities of the body, the condition can be severely aggravated through gas expansion.

Passengers with any of the following should check with their G.P. or M.D. whether they should fly or not. These are high-risk conditions and your doctor may submit a medical information form (M.E.D.I.F.) to the airline's medical department for approval, or may obtain a second opinion from an aviation medical specialist. Do not be surprised if the answer is in the negative, or if it is positive, that you may be required to use supplemental oxygen on board.

Cardiovascular Disease
Angina pectoris. (Occurs when the oxygen supply to the muscle of the heart is impaired.)
Cardiac arrhythmias (unstable). (Disturbances of the heart's rhythm.)
Cerebrovascular accident. (A sudden interruption of the blood supply to the brain.)

Congenital heart disease with poor climatic tolerances. (A heart abnormality existing from birth.)

Congestive failure. (Occurs when the blood vessels or heart becomes clogged with fluid.)

Deep vein thrombosis. (A clot in deep vein.)

High blood pressure. (Severe and pulmonary.)

Myocardial infarction. (An area of dead heart muscle as a result of a blockage of a coronary artery.)

Phlebothrombosis. (Clots in a large vein without inflammation. As a result, there is no pain and the clot might move into the lungs before it is discovered.)

Thrombophlebitis. (Inflammation and clots in a vein.)

Valvular lesions. (Damaged or diseased heart valves.)

Respiratory Diseases

Asthma. (A respiratory disorder characterised by a difficulty in breathing, wheezing and a feeling of constriction in the chest.)

Bronchiectasis. (A chronic enlargement of the bronchial tubes either in length or to form cavities.)

Bronchitis. (Chronic inflammation of the bronchial tubes.)

Bullous lung disease. (Blisters, blebs or bubbles associated with emphysema.)

Congenital pulmonary cyst. (An abnormal swelling containing fluid on the lung existing from birth.)

Cor pulmonale or pulmonary heart disease. (Enlargement of right side of heart caused by chronic lung disease or disorder of pulmonary circulation.)

Emphysema. (The wearing out of the elastic tissue of the lung so that it remains inflated and results in impaired respiration.)

Lobectomy. (The surgical removal of one of the five lobes of the lung.)

Pneumonia. (Infection of the lung in which air pockets or alveoli become filled with liquid and useless for breathing.)

Pneumonectomy. (Surgical removal of a lung or part of a lung.)

Pulmonary embolism. (A clot or air bubble resulting in reduced circulation to the lung.)

Tuberculosis. (A contagious disease caused by infection with tubercle bacteria most frequently affecting the lungs.)

Neurological Conditions

Apoplexy or stroke. (A sudden loss of consciousness often followed by paralysis which is caused by interruption of normal circulation to the brain.)

Atherosclerosis. (Thickening of the inner lining of the arterial walls.)

Brain tumour. (An abnormal swelling in the brain which could be benign or malignant.)

Cerebral infarction. (An area of dead brain tissue.)

Epilepsy. (A disorder characterized by loss of consciousness with or without convulsions.) Epileptics may be more subject to seizures during flight because of a combination of factors such as oxygen lack, hyperventilation, excitement about flying, stress and fatigue.

Mental Illness

Psychosis. (A severe mental disorder.)

Blood Disorders

Anaemia. (Bloodlessness or a deficiency of the oxygen-carrying component, haemoglobin.)

Haemophilia. (A hereditary disease, characterised by impairment or loss of clotting ability of blood.)

Leukaemia. (A disease in which there is a proliferation of white blood corpuscles and suppression of the blood forming function.)

Sickle-cell disease. (A hereditary condition whereby the red blood corpuscles are sickle-shaped.)

Progressive kidney or liver failure.

Gastrointestinal disease

(Expansion of gas in the digestive tract which may cause problems.)

Acute diverticulitis. (Inflammation of a mucous membrane pouch that bulges out through a weak part of the large intestine wall.)

Acute gastroenteritis. (Inflammation of both the stomach and the intestines.) Initial symptoms are nausea, stomach-ache or a feeling of discomfort which is followed by vomiting and diarrhoea. It is usually spread through contaminated food, or the infection may be airborne.

Acute aesophageal varicies. (Varicose veins in the gullet.)

Peptic ulcer or stomach and duodenal ulcer. (An open sore occurring on the mucous membrane of the stomach or on the first part of the duodenum.)

Ulcerative colitis. (A severe persistent inflammation of the colon or large intestine.)

Recent Surgery
Abdominal, chest, ear and facial including wired mandibular fractures.

Pneumothorax
(Air in the space between the lung and the wall of the chest that results in the collapse of the lung.)

Pneumoperitoneum
(Air in the abdominal cavity.)

Unstabilized Convalescent, Post-operative and Handicapped People

Severe Diabetes Mellitus
(A disorder caused by a deficiency of insulin which is characterized by excessive thirst and increased quantities of urine containing an excess of sugar.)

Colostomy or Ileostomy
(A surgical operation to make an artificial opening either for the large intestine – colon or small intestine (ileum).) It may be necessary to vent an increased volume of gastrointestinal gas, so extra

dressings and bags should be taken in the hand luggage.

Large Unsupported Hernia
(The pushing of part of an organ through the wall of a cavity.)

Skull Fracture
(Trapped gas could expand and exert pressure on brain tissue.)

Alcoholism

Korsakoff's Syndrome
(Deterioration of the nerves and brain.)

Delirium Tremens
(A disordered state of mind with hallucinations.)

Infectious Diseases
Anyone with such a disease should not travel, particularly as viruses, bacteria and fungi can be readily spread through the aircraft's ventilation system.

Aviation or Aerospace Medical Specialist

Aviation or aerospace medicine is the preventive specialty that alleviates or protects against the adverse physiological effects caused by the hostile environment of flight. In the U.S., aerospace medicine is a component of the American Board of Preventive Medicine, whereas in the U.K. the Diploma in Aviation Medicine (D AvMed) is insufficient for an Associateship of the Faculty of Occupational Medicine.

The main responsibility of these specialists is as Aviation Medical Examiners of airline pilots who are required by law to have bi-annual medical examinations to hold their licences. Frequent flyers should consider having an annual medical check-up with such a specialist. To obtain the. name of a specialist near you contact the following:

In the U.K.: A list of the medical examiners is supplied in the appendix. Civil Aviation Authority Medical Department, Aviation House, South Area, Gatwick Airport, Gatwick, West Sussex RH6 0YR, tel: 0293 567171 fax: 0293 573999.

In the U.S.: Aerospace Medical Association, 320 S. Henry Street, Alexandria, VA 22314-3524, tel: (703) 739 2240.

Medical Information Form (M.E.D.I.F.)

This form, which is supplied by airlines, is intended to provide confidential information about a passenger to an airline's medical department to assess their fitness to fly. The procedure to follow with a M.E.D.I.F. is given below:

1. Ask your G.P. or physician to complete the form. This will then be submitted to the medical department of the airline with whom you intend to fly for approval.

2. They may give you one of three answers. A. There is no problem for you to travel. B. If you want to travel you will have to do so with supplemental oxygen which is supplied from a portable canister. However, you will be expected to give the airline advance notice of this requirement – at least 48 hours – and there will be a payment for it.

3. You cannot travel by air – it is contra-indicative to your condition – as your life will be at risk.

If you are short of time, go directly to the airline's medical department or to an aviation medical specialist. On the other hand, if you are a frequent flyer, it would be prudent to see a specialist at least once a year. As you may be aware, airline pilots are required by law to have two medical examinations a year to maintain their fitness to fly.

Death In The Clouds

People do die in planes. That is a fact even on the Concorde. These are not deaths of people who would have died anyway but whose deaths have been caused by being in an aircraft.

On a major airline the body bags are brought out once or twice a month. Not much but with greater awareness of aviation medicine (an example of which is given in this book), I am sure those deaths could be avoided in the future. For some sceptical passengers I am quoting two accounts taken from the correspondence column of medical journals. The correspondence column of the first is by Richard Wakeford of Cambridge University of Clinical Medicine.

'We are half-way through the entrée when the call goes out: "If there is a medical doctor on board, would he please make himself known to the cabin staff". A quick glance up and down the cabin expecting to see the usual forest of willing medical and paramedical hands, but no-one responds. The cabin staff look anxious. I put an arm out to a hurrying stewardess and say something tentative like "I'm not a doctor, but if it is a matter of resuscitation then perhaps I can help." "Please come," she says.

'At the back of the aircraft an elderly man, his face an unhealthy colour, is lying on the floor. A stewardess puffs oxygen from a mask towards his face. She is joined by a steward. Together, they start to make a fair attempt at mouth to mouth inflation and external cardiac massage. At the man's head stands another volunteer who looks as uncomfortable as I feel. We exchange credentials. He graduated in medicine from Harvard ten years previously but has never practised medicine. He subsequently qualified as a lawyer. I explain that I am a psychologist who works in medical education research . . .

'We take over inflation and massage. It is messy: the man is incontinent. We ask for medical equipment. A first aid box appears which contains bandages – and a tube, thankfully. The airway clear and the tube inserted, we ask what other medical equipment is available to monitor vital signs. There is none.

'This is Concorde. At twice the speed of sound the noise level is high and the floor vibrates. We can detect no cardiac output but suspect that in these surroundings we never could, even with a stethoscope. We can see no spontaneous breathing. We massage and inflate. Nothing.

'Unqualified to diagnose death and incompetent to do so, I nevertheless have to decide whether to continue – in which case we all go to some Godforsaken spot in eastern Canada – or to stop. We can detect no life. We stop. The aircraft bends towards New York.

'The staff are grateful. No wonder: there are insufficient staff for two of them to spend much time resuscitating passengers, the rest of whom want their coffee and brandy. And the passengers are grateful: Concorde is not going to Goose Bay or wherever. You do not pay £1,400 to be diverted to Goose Bay.

'Emotionally and physically drained, I try ineffectually to clean and tidy the body, but we have not finished. Regulations, we are told, prohibit an aircraft landing with a body in the gangway. "Could you possibly get him back in a seat?" I suggest that this would be inappropriate. So we heave him between the back two rows into the aisle.

'Two armed and bulky New York Port Authority policemen board . . . key witnesses cannot disembark until statements have been taken down. In the terminal I sit exhausted with a beer, awaiting my connection. Has it all happened?

'Better equipment and more fully trained staff might have prevented "my experience" – one that was less characterised by feelings of utter helplessness. They might have enabled us to do a better job. But they would probably not have prevented one of the most harrowing experiences of my life.'

The other account of a death on board comes from Dr J.V. Occleshaw. A female passenger with a history of heart problems, including valve replacements 12 years before, was taken ill on a chartered flight from London to Cyprus.

'Somewhere over Belgium, a call for a doctor came over the passenger address system. I found a stewardess administering oxygen to a very distressed woman. She was clearly in severe left heart failure. It was difficult to be sure that the patient was getting enough oxygen because there was no flow meter and attempts to listen to the gas entering the face mask were frustrated by the noise of the engines. I advised that the patient should be off the aeroplane as soon as possible, and the flight was diverted to a German airport that could be reached in the next 15 minutes.

'The aircraft's medical box contained an ampoule of frumeside with two syringes and needles. After administering the frumeside intravenously, I began to think that the patient might survive, but two minutes later she regurgitated and inhaled her stomach contents. The only equipment available for clearing the airway was a small suction apparatus more suitable for a newborn baby, and suction proved ineffective. The patient's condition deteriorated rapidly and she died. We returned to the airport of departure.

'Charter flights tend to be fully loaded and if there is an in-flight emergency there is nowhere for a patient to be transferred to and treated discreetly. Aircraft cannot, of course, carry a miniature intensive care unit but airways, catheters and a portable battery driven suction apparatus should be provided. A wider range of life-saving drugs should be included in the medical box.'

He concluded that with what it cost in extra fuel to divert back to the airport of departure, the airline could have upgraded all its doctor's kits, including the suction pump which cost £106 and weighed just one kilo.

Post-Flight Deaths

The classic case of a post-flight death is that of the American poet, Robert Lowell. Like most passengers today he was unaware of the link between his health and air travel.

He suffered from congestive heart failure (see High risk conditions, page 58), a condition he described as when 'the lungs filled with water, because the heart can't squeeze enough'. In an aviation medical specialist's casebook, it is contra-indicative to air travel. That does not rule out flying, but it may mean the passenger requires supplemental oxygen on board. To exacerbate matters, Robert Lowell also chain-smoked.

Once William Styron recalled they were both on a 747 and in spite of Lowell requesting a seat in the smoking section, he was placed in a non-smoking one. He 'smoked anyway, much to the annoyance and finally the fury of a non-smoker whose protests to the stewardesses were of no avail. Cal (Robert Lowell) referred to this passenger contemptuously as an "environmentalist!" I was rather tickled by his obstinacy.'

Then he took one trip too many. On September 12, 1977, in the afternoon, he arrived back in New York from Dublin. At Kennedy Airport, he took a taxi into Manhattan. When the driver reached West 67th Street, he noticed that Lowell had slumped in his seat as if he was asleep. He had expired at the age of 60. The next day he was mourned as 'perhaps the best English language poet of his generation'.

How many other people in the world die like that, within hours or a few days of their return flight? Their disease having been tipped into a crisis through exposure to the cabin environment. An unnecessary loss, or in Lowell's words, 'The night dark before its hour'.

Statistics on Medical Incidents

In a world where there is an explosion of statistics, statistical information on medical incidents on board aircraft is a rare exception. There is a dearth of accurate data which is understandable as the airlines play both the gamekeeper and poacher roles by default. No Government legislation compels them to compile statistics nor is there an international body with a mandate to collect objective information. However, there is a legal obligation to register a death as one would expect.

In an important eight-year survey carried out by the International Air Transport Association (I.A.T.A.), a maximum of only 39% of the 120 members participated in any one year. Of the in-flight deaths, 66% were men aged an average of 54 years. But the surprising fact is that 77% of these passengers reported no health problems before departure and more than half died from heart problems. Doctors or physicians, on the other hand, were present at some 43% of the deaths.

Aircraft Doctors

Aircraft, unlike ships, do not have a doctor on board for each flight. This is in spite of the fact that some members of the medical establishment believe that there should be qualified medical help available. However, should an emergency arise, a request for a doctor's assistance is put out on the tannoy. If any are present, some will try to duck out of the responsibility because should they accidentally injure a passenger while offering treatment, they could be sued. There is no 'Good Samaritan' law that is universally applicable.

Should a physician appear, he or she will be given a medical kit and endeavour to deal with the emergency. If this is not possible then the pilot will be asked to divert the aircraft. Sometimes to their chagrin, doctors find that their presence attracts a life-threatening illness much in the same way as an albatross around a boat or ship is said to bring bad luck. On the other hand, if no doctor is present (or they want to remain incognito) an unscheduled landing will be made.

CHAPTER NINE

THE ARMCHAIR
AVIATOR

Once you have found an oasis of calm read the following reflections on flying as they could put you in the right state of mind for your trip:

The Miracle of Flight

All too often we forget how modern aviation is. It is only this century that we began to fly. Before then we had always associated flying with myths, religion or spiritual matters. The heavens were the divine domain of gods or God.

It is not difficult therefore to imagine what happened at this intersection in history. Take the example of a January day in 1910. Some 30,000 eyes at an air meet in Los Angeles focussed on the wheels as they revolved faster and faster and then stopped suddenly when the flying machine rose into the air. The crowd had waited for the miraculous moment and had seen the miracle. In England, this euphoria was tempered by the fear of aviation as a threat to national security. When Bleriot flew across the English Channel, H.G. Wells speculated about a future war that would be fought from the air.

But for at least some two decades, from the Wrights' first flight in 1903 to Lindbergh's triumphant Atlantic crossing in 1927, flying was deemed as being divine and the pilot hailed as a god. American clergymen described Lindbergh's feat as an example of self-control, necessary to 'discipline the flesh' in order to lead the heroic adventure of Christian life. Poems written by the public contained lines such as 'Man is divine, and meant by God to soar!'

This attitude lingered on into the late forties when the U.S. ace and airline executive, Eddie Rickenbacker, observed that pilots had 'always felt inwardly that what they were doing was all part of some mysterious Universal Plan', and they were mere 'pawns of the Creator'.

Gradually, the religious connotation has given way to another worship – that of the plane; a secular religion of the flying machine. It ushered in a new period in human relations and world affairs. Most of the arguments of the day affirmed that a new perspective would be given to mankind. The small petty circumstances in life would pale into insignificance alongside great eternal truths that would become evident.

As we know, the conquest of the skies gave way to the conquest of space and the prophetic creed of the winged gospel preached during those early years was in part realised.

Dreams of Flying

The interpretation of dreams is an age-old pre-occupation. In modern times, there have been professional interpreters like Freud who observed that dreams about flying or birds had a sexual connotation, and Jung, who believed that birds or wings were symbols of spirituality.

Many children have dreams of flying in which they have a sensation of swimming or gliding through the air. This not only enables them to escape from the world they live in but to have out-of-body (O.O.B.) experiences. For example, it is quite common to dream of being killed in a car or plane crash. Once the aircraft bursts into flames or disintegrates, the only feeling they recall is of soaring upwards. There is also the knowledge that they are dead. No pain or panic was experienced. Others tell of leaving their body during sleep and travelling on an 'astral plane' to visit another world. Later, when they return to their body, they usually do so with regret.

The more conventional flying dreams demonstrate travel towards some destination and encountering obstacles on the way. The journey may symbolise the dreamer's life. The destination may represent a lovers' meeting or a death or an arrival at whatever position signifies fulfilment.

Where planes are missed in anxious dreams often represent lost opportunities. When a destination is named eg a westward trip could spell out ageing or death. On the other hand, a trip to Rome could refer to the fact that all thoughts lead to a significant event in your life, like death or love.

The appearance of luggage in dreams usually designates burdens of guilt or responsibilities we carry in life. But depending on the circumstances, such items could also be seen as assets or treasures.

Socrates on Flying in the Universe

In Plato's Phaedrus, Socrates provides an original allegory of the soul, the meaning of life, heaven and hell. Socrates, who died in 399 B.C., projects a remarkable spectacle of gods and some human beings on a flight around our galaxy. On such a great circuit, which will command views outside it, we will find true reality, absolute knowledge and justice.

He begins with the comparison of the soul to a winged charioteer with a team of two horses. One is a thoroughbred while the other is a bad stumpy hybrid. As a result, the task of controlling them is made difficult. The gods, on the other hand, have the best horses and charioteers.

Next Socrates differentiates between mortal and immortal living beings. The soul when it is 'perfect and winged moves on high and governs all creation, but the soul that has shed its wings falls until it encounters solid matter'. There it dons a body and the 'combination of soul and body' is called a human being and is mortal.

How then does the body lose and shed its wings? Before we can answer that question we have to understand its function. The wings lift us into heaven which is inhabited by the gods. Their source of nourishment is 'beauty, wisdom, goodness and every other excellence ... but their opposites such as ugliness and evil cause the wings to waste and perish'.

The soul, which is immortal, explains Socrates, is one that reaches the top of the arch and moves outside the vault to stand on the back of the galaxy. There 'they are carried around by its revolution while they contemplate what lies outside the heavens. But of this region beyond the skies no mortal poet has sung or ever will sing in such strains as it deserves.'

However, we must be truthful about what we see for this is where we find reality. A 'reality without colour or shape, intangible but utterly real, apprehensive only by intellect which is the pilot of the soul. So the mind of a god, sustained as it is by pure intelligence and knowledge, like that of every soul to assimilate its proper food, is satisfied at last with the vision of reality, and nourished and made happy by the contemplation of truth, until the circular revolution brings it back to its starting point.'

During such a journey, absolute justice and absolute knowledge is encountered unlike anything which we have experienced on earth. Once the circuit has been completed, the charioteer withdraws into the vault of heaven and returns home.

There are three types of soul, according to Socrates. The first is able to keep the head of its charioteer above the surface during the circuit in spite of disobedient horses, which at times impair 'its vision of reality'. The second sees only part of the vision of reality because the charioteer sometimes rises and falls below the surface. The third, which comprise the majority, never reach the upper world and move only below the surface 'trampling and jostling one another, each eager to outstrip its neighbour. Great is the confusion and struggle and sweat, and many souls are lamed and many have their wings all broken through the feebleness of their charioteers; finally, for all their toil, they depart without achieving initiation into the vision of reality, and feed henceforth on mere opinion.'

For the first type of soul, it will be free of hurt until the next great circuit with the gods. But for the other souls, who miss the vision, they lose their wings, sink to earth under the burden of forgetfulness and wrong-doing. It takes 10,000 years for a soul to grow its wings again. There are exceptions to the rule. A philosopher, for example, who seeks wisdom without guile can reduce that period.

Poems

There was an American, John Gillespie Magee Jnr, who could not wait to fly in the Second World War. So he joined the Royal Canadian Air Force (R.C.A.F.). He died early on after writing this sonnet, which is revered by pilots of the United States Air Force (U.S.A.F.). It is traditional to give a memento, on which the poem is written, to a colleague whenever he transfers from one assignment to another.

'Oh, I have slipped the surly bonds of earth,
And danced the skies on laughter-silvered
      wings;
Sunward I've climbed, and joined the tumbling
      mirth
Of sun-split clouds – and done a hundred
      things
You have not dreamed of – wheeled and
      soared and swung
High in the sunlit silence. Hov'ring there
I've chased the shouting wind along, and flung
My eager craft through footless halls of air.
Up, up the long, delirious, burning blue
I've topped the windswept heights with easy
      grace
Where never lark, or even eagle flew –
And, while with silent, lifting mind I've trod
The high untrespassed sanctity of space,
Put out my hand, and touched the face of God.'

An Irish Airman Forsees His Death (1917):

> '*I know that I shall meet my fate*
> *Somewhere among the clouds above;*
> *Those that I fight I do not hate*
> *Those that I guard I do not love;*
> *My country is Kiltartan Cross*
> *My countrymen Kiltartan's poor*
> *No likely end could bring them loss*
> *Or leave them happier than before.*
> *Nor law, nor duty bade me fight*
> *Nor public men, nor cheering crowds,*
> *A lovely impulse of delight*
> *Drove to this tumult on the clouds*
> *I balanced all, brought all to mind,*
> *The years to come seemed waste of breath*
> *A waste of breath the years behind*
> *In balance with this life, this death.*'
>
> W.B. Yeats

A poem from a Kamikaze pilot who went on a suicide mission by crashing his plane, a rocket-powered Ohka Kamikaze, into an American ship. The plane carried a 2,645 lb bomb which was more than half its total weight. The Japanese word, 'kami', means divine, and 'kaze' is wind, i.e. divine wind.

Six thousand kamikazes were used during the invasion of Okinawa. It is worth noting that the Japanese consider cherry blossoms as symbolizing dead warriors.

> '*Like cherry blossoms*
> *In the spring,*
> *Let us fall*
> *Clean and radiant.*'
> Heiichi Okabe, aged 22.

DESTINATIONS OF HIGH ALTITUDE

Cities and airports located at high altitude should be more widely known because they prolong the effects of oxygen lack experienced on an aircraft. Not only can these destinations cause mountain sickness, but they can also tip people who have lung, heart or venous disorders into a crisis phase.

I once felt nauseous in Mexico City and wrongly attributed these symptoms to the heat. Had I known any better, I would have taken a couple of days to acclimatize instead of going off sightseeing soon after arrival.

The following list is given (see entry: Mountain Trekking, page 23):

Location	Altitude In Feet
Potisi, Bolivia	13,000
Lhasa, Tibet	12,000
La Paz, Bolivia	11,700
Cuzco, Peru	11,000
Quito, Ecuador	9,200
South Pole Station (U.S.A.)	9,100
Sucre, Bolivia	9,100
Val d'Isere, France	6,600–11,400
Zermatt, Switzerland	5,300–12,500
Toluca, Mexico	8,700
Bogota, Colombia	8,300
Machu Picchu, Peru	8,000
St Moritz, Switzerland	6,000–10,800
Cochabamaba, Bolivia	8,300
Zacatecas, Mexico	8,000
Pachuca de Soto, Mexico	7,900
Addis Ababa, Ethiopia	7,900
Asmara, Ethiopia	7,900
Aspen, Colorado	7,700

Location	Altitude In Feet
Arequipa, Peru	7,500
Mexico City, Mexico	7,500
Netzahualcoyotl, Mexico	7,400
Darjeeling, India	7,400
Sining, Tsinghai, China	7,300
Laramie, U.S.A.	7,200
Sana'a, N. Yemen	7,200
Simla, India	7,200
Puebla, Mexico	7,000
Manizales, Colombia	7,000
Santa Fe, U.S.A.	6,900
Guanajuato, Mexico	6,700
Johannesburg	5,700
Nairobi	5,400

LIST OF APPROVED DOSIMETRY SERVICES

Frequent flyers would be well advised to have their radiation levels checked at a dosimetry laboratory if they fly mainly longhaul and spend an average of 800 hours per year in the air or 400 hours per year on Concorde.

The dosimetry laboratories listed below provide monitoring services for radiation doses and are approved by the Health and Safety Executive.

Addenbrooke's Hospital, Medical Physics Laboratory
Hills Road, Cambridge CB2 2QQ
Approved for: Whole Body Film.

A.E.A. Technology, Radiation Dosimetry Department
Building 364, Harwell Laboratory, Oxfordshire OX11 0RA
Approved for: Whole Body Film & Neutron.

A.E.A. Technology, Winfrith Dosimetry Laboratory
Building A40, Winfrith Technology Centre, Dorchester, Dorset DT2 8DH
Approved for: Whole Body T.L.D. (Thermoluminescent Personal Dosemeters).

Amersham International plc, Amersham Laboratories
White Lion Road, Amersham, Buckinghamshire HP7 9LL
Approved for: Whole Body Film.

British Nuclear Fuels plc, Health Physics & Safety Dept
Chapelcross Works, Annan, Dumfrieshire DG12 6RF
Approved for: Whole Body Film.

British Nuclear Fuels plc, Health Physics &
Safety Dept.
Springfield Works, Salwick, Preston,
Lancashire PR4 0XJ
Approved for: Whole Body Film.

Christie Hospital, Personal Dosimetry Service
Wilmslow Road, Withington,
Manchester M20 9BX
Approved for: Whole Body Film, Extremity.

Landauer, Inc., The Atrium Court
Apex Plaza, Reading,
Berkshire RG1 1AX
Approved for: Whole Body T.L.D.

Leicester Royal Infirmary, District Dept. of
Medical Physics & Clinical Engineering
Leicester LE1 5WW
Approved for: Whole Body Film.

National Nuclear Corp Ltd., Booths Hall
Chelford Road, Knutsford,
Cheshire WA16 8QZ
Approved for: Whole Body T.L.D., Extremity.

N.R.P.B., Scottish Centre
155 Hardgate Road,
Glasgow G51 4LS
Approved for: Whole Body Film.

Nuclear Electric plc, Personal Dosimetry Service
Berkeley Technology Centre, Berkeley,
Gloucestershire GL13 9PB
Approved for: Whole Body Film.

Queen Elizabeth Hospital, Regional Radiation
Physics & Protection Service, Queen Elizabeth
Medical Centre
Edgbaston, Birmingham B15 2TH
Approved for: Whole Body Film, Extremity.

Royal Sussex County Hospital, Brighton Health
Authority, Medical Physics Department,
Radiation Safety Service

Eastern Hospital, Eastern Road,
Brighton BN2 5BE
Approved for: Whole Body Film, Extremity.

Southampton Radiation Service, University of
Southampton, Medical Physics Department,
Centre Block
Southampton General Hospital,
Southampton SO9 4XY
Approved for: Whole Body T.L.D.

Velindre Hospital, Radiation Protection Service
Velindre Road, Whitchurch
Cardiff CF4 7XL
Approved for: Whole Body Film.

Walsgrave Hospital, Department of Clinical
Physics
Radiotherapy Centre, Clifford Bridge Road,
Walsgrave, Coventry CV2 2DX
Approved for: Whole Body Film.

Further advice on radiation can be obtained from
your local Health Authority Radiation Protection
Adviser (R.P.A.) who is usually a medical physi-
cist and supplies a scientific support service to
hospital departments such as X-ray, radiotherapy
and nuclear medicine.

In the U.S.A. there is a National Voluntary Laboratories Accreditation Program (N.A.V.L.A.P.)
organized by the National Institute of Standards
and Technology, Building 235, Room A106,
Gaithersburg, Maryland 20899. Telephone: 301
975 4016. Addresses of dosimetry laboratories can
be obtained from the latter.

Useful Address
Aviation Health Institute
8 King Edward Street, Oxford OX1 4HL
Telephone: 0865 739681
Fax: 0865 726583
The A.H.I. is a medical research charity for
passengers' health. Registered No. 1017574.

CHECKLIST OF VACCINATIONS AND HEALTH PRECAUTIONS

Childhood vaccinations
Diphtheria
Pertussis (whooping cough)
Tetanus: primary course 3 monthly injections.
Boosters every 10 years
Poliomyelitis (live oral or killed injectable) lasts 10 years

Viral hepatitis
Hepatitis A vaccine: 2 injections, 2–4 weeks apart, booster after 6–12 months, lasts 10 years
Normal immunoglobulin lasts 2–6 months, give as late as possible before departure
Hepatitis B (vaccine course six months in advance for anyone coming into contact with human blood) (also sexually transmitted and by contaminated needles)

Rabies (Merieux UK 0628-785291)
Pre-exposure in endemic areas (3 monthly injections in one year) lasts 2 years

Meningococcal meningitis
African meningitis belt (Dec–Feb), New Delhi, Nepal, Mecca
Groups A and C only (single dose) lasts 3 years
Risk in northern Africa, South East Asia, South America, India, Nepal, Middle East

Japanese B (Cambridge Selfcare Diagnostics Ltd 091-261-5950)
Asia only, especially South East Asia, NW

Thailand, Sri Lanka, Nepal, rural areas during and after rains (eg June–Sept)
Three injections 1–2 weeks, 4 weeks, booster after 1 year

Tick borne encephalitis (Immuno Ltd 0732-458101)
Forested areas of Europe and Scandinavia, late spring–summer
Three injections spaced 4–12 weeks, 9–12 months, lasts 3 years

Plague, Anthrax
(High risk area/activity only)

Cholera
In epidemic areas and for certificate: (2 doses, 1–4 weeks) lasts six months (confers only marginal personal protection)

Typhoid
1) Injectable (killed) whole cell vaccine: (2 doses, 4–6 weeks) lasts three years (Evans Medical Ltd 0403-41400)
2) Injectable (killed) Vipolysaccharide vaccine: single dose lasts three years (Merieux UK 0628-785291)
3) Oral (live) vaccine: 1 capsule on alternate days 3 lasts 3 years (Evans Medical Ltd)

Yellow Fever
Affected areas of Africa and South America only. (Live vaccine) (single dose) lasts 10 years, not suitable for those hypersensitive to eggs or with immunosuppression

Tuberculosis
For those with no BCG scar (or record of successful BCG vaccination) who are tuberculin negative, who are not immunosuppressed and do not have eczema.
0.1 ml intradermal BCG

Chemoprophylaxis
Malaria
Traveller's diarrhoea
Typhus
Leptospirosis

Other health precautions
Before departure – dental check, blood group determination (free if you offer to donate blood), generous medical insurance, spare glasses and supply of drugs for chronic diseases (eg diabetes, asthma, rheumatoid arthritis etc).
Anti-mosquito precautions
Needles and syringes (in HIV/hepatitis B endemic areas)
Sun protection
Precautions against mountain sickness if travelling to altitude (depends on target altitude, speed of climb etc)

D.H.S.S. contacts for immunization advice
Birmingham:	021-772-4311
Glasgow:	041-946-7120 (travel prolaxis), extension 277 (for treatments)
Liverpool:	051-708-9393
London:	071-387-4411 (treatment)
	071-388-9600 (travel prolaxis)
	071-636-8636 (travel prolaxis)
	071-636-7921 (recorded advice)
Oxford:	0865-225-570

BIBLIOGRAPHY

Barry, M. and Bia, F. (1989), Pregnancy and travel, Journal of American Medical Association, 261(5): 728–31

Bert, P. (1943), Barometric Pressure, trans. Hitchcock, M.A. and Hitchcock, F.A., Columbus, Ohio: College Book Company

Boeing 747-400 Operations Manual

Dawood, R. (edit.) (1992), Traveller's Health, Oxford: Oxford University Press

DeHart, R. (edit.) (1992), Fundamentals of Aerospace Medicine, Philadelphia, PA: Lea and Febiger

Engle, E. and Lott, A. (1979), Man in Flight, Annapolis, MD: Leeward Publications

Ernsting, J. and King, P. (1988), Aviation Medicine, 2nd Edition, London: Butterworths

Hamilton, I. (1983), Robert Lowell, London: Faber and Faber

Harding, R.M. and Mills, F.J. (1988), Aviation Medicine: articles from the British Medical Journal, London: British Medical Association

Kahn, F.S. (1990), The Curse of Icarus – The health factor in air travel, London: Routledge

Kahn, F.S. (1992), Why flying endangers your health, Santa Fe, NM: Aurora Press

Mallon, B. (1992), Children Dreaming, London: Penguin

Milne, R. (1992), Venous thromboembolism and travel, Journal of the Royal College of Physicians, 26(1): 47–9

National Radiological Protection Board, bulletins and brochures

Occleshaw, J. V. (1991), Medical kits on airliners, Lancet, 337, February 23: 494

Plato (1988), Phaedrus and Letters VII and Letters VIII, trans. Hamilton, W., London: Penguin

Rycroft, C. (1991), The innocence of dreams, London: Hogarth Press

Thorn, J. (edit.) (1983), The Armchair aviator, New York: Charles Scribner's Sons

Wakeford, R. (1986), Death in the clouds, British Medical Journal, 293, December 20:1642–3

Weatherall, D.J., Ledingham, J.G.G. and Warrell, D.A. (eds.), Oxford Textbook of Medicine, Oxford: Oxford University Press

INDEX

A
A.I.D.S., 22, 47
aerophobia *see* fear
aerospace medical specialists, 61–2, 76–8
air
  quality, 8–10
  within body, 6–8
air conditioning, 13–14, 15–17
aircraft cabins, 13–14
airline club lounges, 50–1
airports, 49–50
  high altitude, 74–5
alcohol, 30, 43, 53
altitudes
  of aircraft, 13
  of airports, 74–5
anxiety, 25
aromatherapy, 22, 44
aviation medical specialists, 61–2, 76–8

B
baths, 56
Bert, Paul, and airsickness, 3–4
beta-blockers, 30
blood disorders, 59
body bullets, 51
books, for nervous flyers, 32–3
Boyle's Law, 4
breathing, 25–6
  hyperventilation, 17–18, 25
bumping, 55–6

C
carbon dioxide levels, 15–16
cardiovascular disease, 57–8
children, 21, 31
clothing, 31, 54
coffee, 43
colostomy, 60–1
Concorde, 13, 19

contact lenses, 22
contagious diseases, 16, 21–22, 46–7
contraceptive pill, 20
convalescence, 60
courses, for nervous flyers, 32–3
crash survival, 30–2

D
death, 62–6
decompression, 14–15
decompression sickness, 19
dehydration, 8–9
delerium tremens, 61
diabetes, 19, 60
diarrhoea, 46
diet, for jetlag avoidance, 44 *and see* food
diving, 19
doctors, on aircraft, 67 *and see* aviation medical
   specialists
dosimetry services, 76–8
dreams, of flying, 69–70

E
ears, 7, 22, 25
epilepsy, 19, 59
exercise, 43

F
fear, 24–33
flying
   books on, 32–3
   history of, 68–72
   mechanics of, 27–9
   noises made during, 29–30
food, 42–3, 52–3
food hygiene, 46–7
fruit, 52–3

G
gastrointestinal disease, 59–60

H
Hepatits A, 46
hernias, 61
high risk conditions, 57–61
humidity, 8–9, 41
hyperventilation, 17–18, 25 *and see* breathing

hypoxia, 5–6

I
I.U.D.s, 20
ileostomy, 60–1
immune system, 47–8
immunization, 45–6, 48
infectious diseases, 16, 21–22, 46–7, 61

J
jetlag, 34–7
jetlag avoidance, 44, 56
   airwise method, 36–43

K
Korsakoff's Syndrome, 61

L
lucky charms, 26–7

M
malaria, 22, 46
medical check-ups, 25, 61–2
   dosimetry services, 76–8
Medical Information Form (M.E.D.I.F.), 57, 62
medication, 18–19
mental illness, 59
Mile High Club, 32
Moro reflex, 24

N
neurological conditions, 59
noises, from the aircraft, 29–30

O
operations, 60
over-breathing *see* hyperventilation
oxygen, 5–6, 9–10, 41
ozone levels, 16

P
pacemakers, 51
periods, 20
personality changes, 21
pillows, 54
planning, 55–6
plaster casts, 7

poetry, 72–3
pregnancy, 12, 30–1
pressure, 4, 13

R
radiation, 10–12
reading, 26
relaxation, 41, 49–51
respiratory diseases, 58–9

S
safety drills, 31–2
sex, 32
sick aircraft syndrome, 15–17
sinuses, 7, 22
skin conditions, 22–23
skull fractures, 61
sleep, 41
smoke hoods, 31
smoking, 9–10
Socrates, and flying, 70–2
speeds, 13
statistics, medical incidents on board aircraft,
    66–7
stop-offs, 55
stressors, 3, 49, 55
surgery, 7, 60

T
talismans, 26–7
talking, 27
tea, 43
Teddy, 26
teeth, 6
tranquillisers, 30
tuberculosis, 22, 59

U
Unexpected events, 55–6

V
vaccination, 45–6
Valsalva manoeuvre, 22
visas, 54–5

W
water, 41, 53, *and see* humidity